Baking
Soda
for Health

Baking Soda
for Health

100 Amazing and Unexpected Uses for Sodium Bicarbonate

Britt Brandon, CFNS, CPT

Adams Media
New York London Toronto Sydney New Delhi

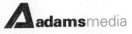

Adams Media
An Imprint of Simon & Schuster, Inc.
57 Littlefield Street
Avon, Massachusetts 02322

First Adams Media trade paperback edition MARCH 2018

ADAMS MEDIA and colophon are trademarks of Simon and Schuster.

For information about special discounts for bulk purchases, please contact Simon & Schuster Special Sales at 1-866-506-1949 or business@simonandschuster.com.

The Simon & Schuster Speakers Bureau can bring authors to your live event. For more information or to book an event contact the Simon & Schuster Speakers Bureau at 1-866-248-3049 or visit our website at www.simonspeakers.com.

Manufactured in the United States of America

10 9 8 7 6 5 4 3 2 1

Library of Congress Cataloging-in-Publication Data
Brandon, Britt, author.
Baking soda for health / Britt Brandon, CFNS, CPT.
Avon, Massachusetts: Adams Media, 2018.
Series: For health.
Includes index.
LCCN 2017055481 (print) | LCCN 2017055989 (ebook) | ISBN 9781507206577 (pb) | ISBN 9781507206584 (ebook)
LCSH: Naturopathy--Popular works. | Sodium bicarbonate--Therapeutic use--Popular works. | BISAC: HEALTH & FITNESS / Alternative Therapies. | HEALTH & FITNESS / Healing. | HEALTH & FITNESS / Beauty & Grooming.
LCC RZ440 (ebook) | LCC RZ440 .B6457 2018 (print) | DDC 615.238222--dc23
LC record available at https://lccn.loc.gov/2017055481

ISBN 978-1-5072-0657-7
ISBN 978-1-5072-0658-4 (ebook)

CONTENTS

Part 2: Beauty 67

INTRODUCTION

What if I told you I could give you a "solve-all" product that could fix almost any issue from athlete's foot and body odor to treating laundry stains and cleansing the refrigerator—*and* it only costs less than ten cents per ounce? Would you be interested? This product is not only real, but you probably have it in your home right now: it's baking soda.

Baking soda is a natural, nontoxic ingredient that can work magic in the kitchen, in the home, or outdoors. Not only is this product easy to use, safe around children, and adaptable to almost any situation or treatment application imaginable, it is also inexpensive and available at almost any location.

For more than one hundred years, consumers have used baking soda in a myriad of ways that include everything from auto care to baking and beauty care. With a simple tablespoon of this product, you can create a detoxifying face mask or grease-eliminating car wash. What makes baking soda so powerful is its grit (when used as a paste), its ability to dissolve into any liquid solution, and its ability to neutralize everything from odor to grease.

Baking Soda for Health will share one hundred uses for baking soda, from soothing upset stomachs and treating acne to tenderizing meat and cleaning up pet accidents. With this book you can use baking soda to transform the health of your home and body naturally and inexpensively. From bathroom cleansers, weed repellent, and even deodorant and beauty masks, you can harness the natural powers of baking soda for limitless benefits! Consumable and absorbable, this nontoxic ingredient can be added to food or used for cleaning…all while promoting your health safely and naturally.

While it may sound funny that the same product can be used in beauty treatments *and* cleaning applications, you'll learn how the neutralizing capabilities of this simple product can safely combat everything from oily skin and acne to rust and mildew. If you're ready to take a chance on an inexpensive product that can help your health and your home, then read on to discover the wonders of baking soda.

BAKING SODA'S MANY HEALTH BENEFITS

With plentiful products that promise to deliver exceptional health and beauty results appearing on late-night infomercials, throughout store shelves, and on various online venues each and every day, it can be difficult to determine which ones are actually able to deliver on their promises and help you better the areas of your body and life that you're striving to improve. While these new and exciting products claim to provide the perfect solution to your issues, they are more likely to fall flat than follow through. Rather than opting for the latest and greatest products that can leave you feeling let down and out of patience, you can choose to utilize an age-old ingredient that has been used by cultures in every country for thousands of years…with success! Baking soda is an ingredient that has been used for an astounding number of years and continues to grace the homes of millions of people around the world for purposes you may have never even considered. When this simple product is sprinkled on food, included in a beauty application, or applied in a cleansing solution that is safe and nontoxic for both humans and pets, baking soda can be a life-changing improvement that is faster, easier, and safer than other alternatives. This book contains one hundred uses that can help you transform your health, your beauty regimen, and your overall quality of life with easy applications of baking soda…the same ingredient you use in your cookies, store in your fridge, and sprinkle on your clothes. While this age-old household staple seems unassuming and quaint, the applications detailed on the following pages will show you how a simple box of powder can help you improve almost every imaginable area of your life…safely and naturally.

What Is Baking Soda?

Baking soda has been commonplace in many homes for many years, and the product is easily identifiable by most people around the world. A majority of consumers have used the powdery product for baking and cooking. The starchy white powder is identified by scientists and chemists with a number of names, such as sodium bicarbonate, sodium hydrogen carbonate, and sodium acid carbonate. The chemical makeup of this multipurpose product is what makes it such a versatile solution to a vast number of cleaning, health, and beauty problems. Baking soda has a pH of 8.1 (neutral pH is 7) and is able to neutralize both acids *and* bases. This type of product is known in scientific terms as "amphoteric." Baking soda can improve the balance of countless solutions including neutralizing bitter tastes in baked goods and cleaning up acid spills in scientific labs.

Nontoxic, harmless, and virtually free of any overdose or exposure risks, this unassuming powder has the capability to solve almost any problem from soothing heartburn and improving blood pressure to deodorizing carpets and cleaning acid spills. Versatility is, without a doubt, the most surprising aspect of baking soda.

BAKING SODA VERSUS BAKING POWDER

While mentioning the common inclusion of baking soda in cooking and baking, it should be noted that "baking soda" and "baking powder" are not the same thing. Baking soda is used in the production of baking powder, but baking powder requires additional ingredients (usually cream of tartar and starch) to be properly formulated.

The History of Baking Soda

Before modern baking soda, the use of "natron" (a naturally occurring mineral salt that contains about 17 percent sodium bicarbonate) was utilized by the ancient Egyptians as far back as 2500 B.C. for everything from food preservation to mummification. In fact, this natural compound was mined around the world by many cultures from deposits that had formed following extensive evaporation of the great salt lakes in Egypt, Venezuela, Kenya, central Asia, and Wyoming. Pure sodium bicarbonate (modern baking soda) didn't start to become a reality until 1791 when a French chemist named Nicolas Leblanc developed a process to mass-produce sodium carbonate, one of the chemical components of baking soda. However, it was another fifty years before John Dwight and his brother-in-law, Austin Church, began mass-producing baking soda in the United States for cooking, cleaning, and household use, developing the first distributing company for the product that would later be known as Arm & Hammer. Throughout the early 1900s, baking soda grew in popularity for its versatility—helping with everything from baking and removing grease, to cleaning laundry and removing odors. From the historic mines of the great salt lakes to refrigerators around the world today, baking soda has evolved and grown in popularity because of its natural ability to cleanse and purify without toxicity, chemicals, or unhealthy additives.

NO ALUMINUM

There is a common misconception that baking soda contains aluminum. This misconception is often perpetuated by certain brands of baking soda that label themselves as "aluminum-free." The truth is baking soda does not contain any aluminum, it is actually baking *powder* that can contain aluminum.

How to Use Baking Soda…for Almost Anything

As baking soda evolved through the years, the product's use expanded to include countless applications. From bakers utilizing the ingredient as a leavening agent to cooks blanching vegetables in water mixed with baking soda to help retain their vibrant colors, the kitchen was where baking soda first became a true necessity. While baking soda can be used for cooking and baking, the powdery substance can also be used in the home for removing odors, treating stains, mild disinfecting, pest control, and removing grease and grime. Incredibly, the same simple powder can be ingested regularly to provide astounding health benefits that can naturally transform a person's well-being. When it was determined that baking soda is water-soluble, the product was used to treat medical conditions such as acidosis, alkalosis, hyperkalemia, indigestion, and heartburn. Soon the medical community started incorporating baking soda into treatment solutions for managing depression, improving blood pressure, minimizing the effect of sodium on hypertension, and (of course) treating gastrointestinal issues resulting from acid-related conditions. Today, the same unassuming box of baking soda that graces your refrigerator door has the power to remove smells from carpets and closets, help baked goods achieve perfection, neutralize bitter tastes in cooked meals, and safely remove grit and grime. Baking soda can also be used in do-it-yourself beauty applications. Incorporating this simple ingredient into your everyday life can provide you with inexpensive, time-saving solutions that can do everything from safely clean your home to help boost your heart health.

Safety Precautions

Baking soda has a slightly salty taste and an alkalizing effect in culinary creations. Having been used successfully for years in applications too numerous to count, the only necessary precaution when handling baking soda is to keep your eyes well protected to prevent irritation resulting from baking soda or any other substance entering them. If baking soda does get in your eyes, it is recommended that you flush your eyes with water for several minutes and then see your doctor.

Of course, you should never use baking soda for a medical application without first checking with your doctor. Also, baking soda should not be given to children under the age of six without first consulting a pediatrician. Beyond those few caveats, baking soda can be used safely and effectively in the treatment of wounds, irritations, inflammation, soreness, and much more!

SAFETY PRECAUTIONS

Baking soda is safe to take internally, but as you will see in the entries in this book, the baking soda should always be completely dissolved in water first before ingesting it. Also, you should not ingest baking soda when you are full. People with kidney disease, high blood pressure, or heart disease should be cautious when taking baking soda because of the high sodium content.

PART 1

HEALTH

Whether you're simply trying to utilize natural ingredients to improve your health or you're concerned about your health because of the onset of a serious condition, baking soda can help. From alleviating ulcer pain to promoting cancer prevention, the simple addition of this easily accessible item can transform your life! For the minimal cost of ten cents, you can improve the health benefits of your salads and smoothies or relieve your pets of their bad breath. Without any concern over the health-compromising chemicals and ingredients that are frequently added to mass-marketed products, you can treat your own health and the health of your home with peace of mind. This first section will discuss the many health-related topics that can be treated with safe, all-natural baking soda. From joint pain to patio weeds, you can use baking soda and the tips and tools in the following entries to make life better. There's no need to be concerned about toxicity or poisoning; these health applications for baking soda can improve your everyday life…naturally and inexpensively.

1: IMPROVES DIGESTIVE SYSTEM FUNCTIONING

When digestive disruptions wreak havoc on your body, everything from eating to sleeping can become complicated. Millions of patients seek relief from digestive system malfunctions every year, and in response, pharmaceutical companies have flooded the market with products that promise to provide relief. Whether you're dealing with acid reflux issues, constipation, or chronic stomach upset, incorporating these products into your daily routine can be more detrimental to your health than you could imagine. Many of these medications contain questionable ingredients and harsh chemicals that can actually worsen conditions or exacerbate pre-existing conditions.

In an effort to avoid the complications associated with these common medications, consumers who are seeking natural digestive system improvement are finding success with the use of baking soda. One teaspoon of baking soda dissolved in an 8-ounce glass of water can be consumed every morning to help maintain a healthy pH balance throughout the digestive system for optimal digestion, minimized acid reflux, and healthy bowel functioning.

This simple solution is safe to consume at any point in the day, and its consumption can not only improve your everyday digestive system functioning, but it can also provide relief for the sudden onset of digestive system upsets that threaten to interfere with daily life. Using this simple solution can not only safeguard your digestive health from pH-related issues, chronic digestive conditions, and serious digestive disease, but it can also improve your overall health and help you maintain that health each and every day.

NATURAL METHODS FOR PREVENTING AND ALLEVIATING DIGESTIVE ISSUES

With the pharmaceutical companies making billions of dollars annually from physicians writing prescriptions for patients suffering from digestive disruptions, the effective natural treatments available are far less promoted and publicized. With all-natural elements such as apple cider vinegar, gingerroot, and baking soda, the body's systems can better regulate the enzymes and metabolic processes involved in digestion to ensure proper digestive system functioning and overall health!

2: IMPROVES CIRCULATORY SYSTEM HEALTH

It takes only a few minutes watching commercials or reading advertisements to hear about the countless medications and prescriptions available that treat issues related to the circulatory system. Arteries, circulation, fatty deposits in the blood stream, and so much more are all promised to be treated with questionable and concerning modern medicines. But, what if there was an all-natural alternative that could help?

The circulatory system is responsible for countless functions throughout the body, including delivering life-sustaining blood, oxygen, and hormones to our vital organs. The circulatory system not only sustains the body, but it also determines our overall level of health. When the circulatory system is compromised, the detrimental consequences can impact daily functions such as energy production, mental function, thought processes, digestion, and immunity. Circulatory issues can lead to the possibility of serious health conditions such as heart disease, chronic respiratory disease, and the development of various blood issues. As a result, many physicians are instructing patients to make an extra effort to focus on circulatory system health by adopting healthy lifestyle habits, eating a heart-healthy diet, and minimizing risks that can directly affect the circulatory system.

While many people have started paying more attention to their heart health, there is a growing majority of health-conscious consumers who are choosing to seek out all-natural alternatives to medications and medical treatments for improving heart health. Baking soda has become an increasingly popular option for cleansing the blood and improving circulatory system performance. Helping to maintain a healthy pH, 1 teaspoon of baking soda dissolved in an 8-ounce glass of water can naturally revitalize the body, improve blood flow, detoxify the blood, and help break down blockages. Baking soda is an excellent and effective all-natural option for improving the health of the circulatory system while also improving overall health and daily life.

3: BOOSTS IMMUNITY

When the immune system is compromised, the results can be disastrous. The quality and health of the immune system can play a major role in determining overall quality of life. Disruptions in everyday life that impact your appetite, energy level, and sleep patterns can lead to serious complications in metabolism, cognitive function, and even the performance of organs and systems. When your immunity is poor, illnesses and conditions can be contracted easily, making every cold and flu season a threat to your body and life. Missing work, not enjoying activities, and having to quarantine yourself away from loved ones are just the tip of the iceberg of falling ill. Something as simple as the common cold can quickly escalate into a serious illness such as pneumonia and become catastrophic.

Medical professionals and holistic healers all agree that the best medicine is prevention, and when you care for your immune system, the results are reflected in how often you succumb to illness and disease. With the addition of baking soda to your everyday routine, you can see an improvement in energy levels, feel less muscle soreness following activity, and experience a better digestive system that seemingly speaks to you about what you should and shouldn't put in your body. Helping to balance the hormones, improve the pH of the blood, and support the healthy functioning and protection of the cells and organs, 1 teaspoon of baking soda dissolved in 1 cup of water can improve immunity and safeguard the health of your body and the quality of your life naturally.

IMMUNITY ASSAILANTS

With questionable ingredients in foods, toxins in the environment, and sicknesses that are ever-present regardless of season, it's no wonder that people suffer from compromised immune system issues regularly. With the implementation of all-natural ingredients such as baking soda, apple cider vinegar, aloe vera, ginger, and turmeric, anyone can help safeguard their immunity (and, thus, their overall health) naturally throughout the year.

4: INCREASES RESPIRATORY SYSTEM'S AIRWAY FUNCTIONING

When most people think of the respiratory system, they tend to think of only the lungs, airways, and the anatomical elements that help us breathe. The truth is that the respiratory system is an intricate part of the body's function to provide and sustain life, but most of us only think of it when a cold, cough, or breathing condition develops.

Every time you take a breath, your lungs fill with air and oxygen is extracted for use in all of your body's other systems, including the heart and the brain. When the respiratory system is not functioning normally, the blood becomes less saturated with essential oxygen, and the body's systems that depend on efficient respiratory functions start to diminish in productivity. When airways and lung capacity become threatened or compromised, the possibility of developing serious conditions such as sinus infections, respiratory infections, COPD (chronic obstructive pulmonary disease), and more increases, causing not only a threat to overall health but also to your lifestyle (especially if an ailment becomes chronic and consistent).

With the inclusion of baking soda in your everyday routine, you can help rid your airways of mold, mildew, spores, and pathogens that can result in chronic agitation and disruption in normal respiratory activity. One teaspoon of baking soda dissolved in an 8-ounce glass of water, combined with ¼ teaspoon of apple cider vinegar improves the health of the metabolic processes that contribute to lung function, opens airways, rids the system of harmful elements, and promotes productive breathing without medications! This tonic can be consumed daily, even when the sudden onset of a respiratory or sinus infection occurs, helping you maintain and safeguard the health of your respiratory system safely and naturally.

5: BENEFITS THE SKELETAL SYSTEM

In order to maintain a healthy skeletal system, the body has to have adequate nutrition. In addition to the essential vitamins and minerals that are required for the body to sustain the health of its bones, the other nutrients that are required by the body also have to be obtained so that the body doesn't turn to the existing nutrients in the bones to satisfy its everyday needs. While many people feel confident about their bone health because of their daily calcium supplementation, the truth is that it may not be enough. Following injury, illness, or the onset of disease, the body relies heavily on calcium and supportive minerals to retain and sustain its mass of bones. Without adequate supplies, these calcium stores become depleted and the bones become brittle, leading to chronic conditions such as osteoporosis, osteoarthritis, and so on. By choosing a calcium-rich diet, exercising regularly, and eliminating harmful habits from everyday life, you can help your body absorb and build bone strength…and baking soda can be another healthy addition.

With baking soda's ability to balance pH naturally, the digestive system becomes increasingly proficient at absorbing the micronutrients (vitamins and minerals) that are necessary to maintaining bone health. With this maximized ability to absorb, distribute, and store micronutrients, the body is able to build and sustain bone health for an extended duration of time, not just the present day. By focusing on the future health of bones, the natural deterioration of bone mass that leaves countless people over the age of fifty vulnerable to fractures, breaks, and in need of major surgeries will not be a concern, and your bones will be healthy enough to sustain falls and accidents without serious incident or injury. One teaspoon of baking soda can be dissolved into an 8-ounce glass of water and consumed daily to ensure that the body's systems are able to function properly, absorb and store nutrients, and maximize the potential for bones not only today, but in the future as well.

6: MINIMIZES ARTHRITIS

Every year, millions of people around the world wake up to the painful symptoms of arthritis. Stiffness, redness, aching joints, and decreased range of motion are just a few of the battles that arthritis sufferers endure each day. This condition has led pharmaceutical companies to create countless prescription and over-the-counter medications that promise to relieve arthritis pain, but often fall flat and also leave the arthritic consumer with additional side effects and complications. Because age, injuries, illnesses, and heredity all play a role in the development, persistence, and intensity of arthritis, most medical professionals advise patients that recovery may be limited but can be improved with healthy lifestyle changes related to diet and exercise. While avoiding specific foods such as nightshade vegetables while implementing daily cardio workouts can be helpful, arthritis sufferers are often left seeking other natural forms of pain relief that don't require pills and potions.

Baking soda can succeed where other medications and applications fall short. By reducing inflammation naturally, improving the body's pH levels, and minimizing the distress on the systems that directly affect the body's ability to maintain proper stores of nutrients, baking soda acts as a defender against the underlying sources of inflammation that contribute to arthritis discomfort. Breaking down the physical complications that contribute to the development of arthritic symptoms, baking soda can not only alleviate symptoms but also assist in the reparation of tissues, cartilage, and inflammatory subsets that result from the condition. With 1 teaspoon of baking soda dissolved in an 8-ounce glass of water, anyone suffering from arthritis pain can find relief naturally, not just for today but for the future as well.

7: ASSISTS IN WOUND HEALING

When a wound occurs, the first thoughts should be to immediately clean it and take care to avoid infection. While people have long considered peroxide the most effective cleaning agent for wounds, it's now known that this go-to agent for wound care actually inhibits the repair of skin tissue. While wounds vary in their severity, consistent care is what helps ensure proper healing without risking infection or permanent damage. While antibiotic wound strips and bandages promise to provide relief from pain and assist in healing, there are all-natural alternatives that can help keep wounds clean, clear of infections, and promote the healing processes that the body undergoes naturally; one of the safest of these alternatives is baking soda. Baking soda is an all-natural alternative that not only helps protect against infection but also improves the body's immune system, reparative capabilities, and abilities to regenerate the tissues and skin as the wound heals.

With an application of a baking soda soak, a wound can be wrapped immediately afterward, helping to rid the wound of harmful bacteria that can cause infection. This application can be made quickly and easily with a paper towel soaked in a solution of equal parts water and baking soda. Following the initial application of the soak, a paste of 1 tablespoon of baking soda and 1 teaspoon of water can be applied to the wound and held in place with a bandage for 10–15 minutes per session, as often as necessary. Not only does this application ensure that the wound remains protected against infiltrating illnesses, but it also promotes the regeneration of skin cells in a safe, pH-balanced environment. With regular changes of the application every 4–6 hours, this protective baking soda wound application has been found to be effective even in severe cases.

ALOE'S EXCEPTIONAL EPIDERMAL EFFECTS

A fun fact about aloe vera is that this natural product helps deliver any ingredient that's added to it below the epidermal surface naturally. When pH-balancing baking soda is combined with aloe vera, both ingredients provide benefits beneath the topical layers of the skin and deliver their nutrients and benefits throughout the skin's layers. Without risking safety or skin irritation, these ingredients promote simple, fast, and effective healing that simultaneously contributes to the health of the skin.

8: IMPROVES NERVOUS SYSTEM FUNCTIONING

Most people don't consider the extreme importance of the optimal functioning of the nervous system. The nervous system controls your sight, hearing, taste, smell, and touch sensations. It is also in charge of your movement and balance, helps with blood flow and blood pressure, and is essential in your ability to think. The nervous system is comprised of your brain and spinal cord (your central nervous system) and the nerves in your body that control your voluntary and involuntary movements (your peripheral nervous system).

With an adequately supported nervous system, everything from the brain's cognitive processes to the muscles' ability to perform daily activities is able to perform as designed. Despite how pivotal this system is, it's surprising that countless patients with issues associated with nervous system dysfunction aren't aware of the importance of daily care dedicated to improving and supporting this area of health.

Eating a balanced, low-fat diet with ample supplies of vitamins B_6, B_{12}, and folate will help protect your nervous system, as will drinking plenty of water, exercising regularly, getting rest, and quitting smoking. By making an effort to focus on nervous system health, patients not only improve their range of motion, cognitive function, and endurance, but also see an unexpected improvement in other areas of their lives, including quality of focus, memory, sleep, endurance, and body temperature regulation. Without the nervous system being supported with adequate supplies of vitamins and minerals, these areas of life suffer and diminish, but baking soda can help in an unexpected way.

By improving the pH of the body, 1 teaspoon of baking soda dissolved in an 8-ounce glass of water interacts with unhealthy enzymes, bacteria, and fluids that can inhibit the absorption of essential nutrients. Baking soda also promotes the nervous system's ability to repair and regenerate damaged cells and nerves.

9: ASSISTS IN IMPROVING REPRODUCTIVE HEALTH

Every year, countless couples struggle to achieve successful conception. Sadly, many of these men and women strive to live the healthiest lives possible in order to bring a child into this world… to no avail. Hormonal imbalance, pH imbalance, ovulation irregularities, and inadequate sperm production or mobility are some of the most commonly known conditions that can interfere with reproductive health. Many hopeful future parents turn to medical professionals for one of the many medical and procedural options that promise to increase the chances of conception, but these options can wreak havoc on the body and mind. These medications, prescriptions, and procedures can do irreparable damage to the body's cells, organs, and systems, leaving patients who are seeking to conceive considering all-natural alternatives. By making healthy lifestyle changes that include reduced red meat consumption, avoidance of antibiotics, and an improvement in healthy lifestyle habits, such as exercise, adequate vitamin and mineral consumption, and adequate sleep, couples have seen drastic improvements in fertility.

In addition, daily doses of baking soda by both male and female partners can help the body reduce or rid itself of inhibiting elements that interfere with hormone production, nutrient absorption and distribution, and circulation of blood to the sex organs. One teaspoon of baking soda dissolved in an 8-ounce glass of water can not only regulate pH and provide the body with health-improving benefits that help in the process of conception, but it can also assist in the healing of other underlying conditions.

NATURAL FERTILITY PROMOTION

Each year, countless individuals and couples seek treatment for infertility. With a few lifestyle changes (dietary improvements, eliminating alcohol and tobacco products, and adopting a regular exercise program), simple, natural additions like baking soda can make a major improvement in overall health that can promote natural fertility and prepare for a healthy pregnancy naturally.

10: RELIEVES INSECT BITES

If you've ever endured the painful intensity of a bug bite, then you can identify with the desperate quest for relief. Whether the itch is isolated to a single spot or causing your body to break out in hives, the physical symptoms resulting from a bug bite can be life-altering: disrupted sleep; nausea; and even inhibited mental focus, cognitive awareness, and memory. Many over-the-counter applications promise to provide relief from these "minor" irritations. In fact, it can seem easy to simply breeze through your favorite grocery store or drug store, purchase a tube or spray bottle of insect-bite reliever, and handle the situation without another thought. However, the application of these seemingly innocent medications can actually cause more harm than good. With dangerous chemical ingredients and preservatives that can cause serious irritation, over-the-counter insect-bite relievers should be considered possible irritants rather than products to soothe an irritated, infected, or open wound.

Baking soda, on the other hand, can be utilized in a number of applications that prevent irritation, soothe itchiness, reduce inflammation, and relieve redness. Ingesting 1 teaspoon of baking soda dissolved in an 8-ounce glass of water will help soothe bites by promoting healing processes from the inside out. In addition, a one-to-one ratio of baking soda and aloe vera can be soaked into a compress and applied to the site of the bite directly several times a day for immediate relief, protection, and promotion of healing.

WORKS FOR PETS TOO

If your pet has an insect bite that is causing him discomfort, you can also use baking soda topically on his bite. Simply mix 1 teaspoon of baking soda with a bit of water to form a paste and apply it to the sting. Try to leave it on for at least 15 minutes if your pet will allow this. The baking soda will provide a cooling effect and will help neutralize the acid of the bite.

11: SOOTHES STINGS

When you're suffering from the pain, inflammation, and redness that takes hold of the skin as a result of a sting, the irritation can almost seem as if it affects your mind as much as your body. The venom and poison that gets deposited in the bloodstream after a sting can cause everything from mild symptoms of pain at the site to major symptoms such as blurred vision and nausea. Stings often vary in discomfort levels because biological composition and makeup can vary from one person to the next, making each person's physical reaction to stings vary widely. With most insect stings, though, sudden onset of immediate pain and inflammation are to be expected.

Seemingly simple sting-relieving applications that can be purchased over the counter can be questionable in terms of their effectiveness and their composition. Baking soda, on the other hand, will not only provide a sting sufferer with relief, but will also speed healing time, improve the irritated area's inflammatory response, and reduce redness. By soaking a cloth with water, sprinkling the stung area with 1 teaspoon of baking soda, and holding the compress in place for 30–45 minutes after the sting, relief can be felt immediately, increasing and improving the healing process naturally.

While stings can feel awful on the skin's surface, many people have physical reactions internally, such as anaphylactic shock, that can be far more serious. Ingesting 1 teaspoon of baking soda in an 8-ounce glass of water can help purge venom from the bloodstream, return the pH levels of the body back to normal, and reduce the impact of the foreign venom drastically, continuing to do so over extended time periods. By using this combination of ingested and topical baking soda, anyone can find relief from a sting safely, easily, and naturally.

12: REMOVES SPLINTERS

Few people realize that the difficulty in extracting a splinter is all based on the body's physical response to an irritant entering the skin's surface. When a splinter enters into the skin, the body's immediate reaction is to become inflamed and try to push the foreign object out naturally. Ironically, this natural response can trap the splinter in the swelled skin and make it difficult to extract.

When trying to remove a splinter from the skin, many people attempt the extraction with tweezers, only to find that the inflammation has already trapped the foreign substance in the skin. Once the initial attempt to simply remove the splinter fails, the need to utilize tools such as needles, pins, or even scalpels can seem imminent. However, using unsterilized tools to enter the skin's surface to retrieve a splinter can introduce countless bacteria into the body and cause infection. Once this occurs, the site of the splinter becomes far more irritated and inflamed…possibly leading to a major assault on the immune system.

Making a soak that is comprised of 1 part baking soda and 4 parts water (for example, 1 cup of water and ¼ cup of baking soda) results in a simple solution that can be made and used to soak the afflicted area that holds the splinter, reducing the inflammation, and naturally assisting the body in pushing the splinter out of the skin. This soak can also help safeguard the affected area from infection by bacteria and microbes that entered the open wound's surface. Naturally and effectively, this is the safest approach to removing splinters without damaging the skin or the body's immune systems or processes.

13: ALLEVIATES ULCERS

Every year, millions of people are diagnosed with ulcers and ulcer-related conditions. Suffering from symptoms such as heartburn, upset stomachs, diarrhea, and "lightning-like" shooting pains that react to the digestion of any food or liquid, an ulcerative patient can face excruciating pain every day. While everything consumed is meant to be digested properly with the help of countless digestive fluids and enzymes that are ever present in the digestive system, there are a number of conditions that can cause these fluids to work against the body and contribute to the deterioration of the lining of the colon. Whether the condition is related to stress, consumption of medication, or inadequate pH levels, the development of an ulcer can lead to indescribable discomfort, pain, and a disruption of everyday life activities.

While there are countless medications available that promise to provide relief for ulcer-related conditions, these medications (both over-the-counter and prescription) can contain harsh chemicals and additives that do more harm than good, leaving patients with side effects that can cause irreparable damage to the brain and body.

Baking soda provides ulcer patients with a healthy alternative that is not only effective in repairing damage to the systems in which the ulcer has developed but also in maintaining proper pH balance and restoring digestive health for future prevention of ulcerative development. One teaspoon of baking soda dissolved in 1 cup of water can help maintain healthy functioning of all systems while preventing, repairing, and restoring the body's dysfunctions related to ulcers.

ULCER PAIN

Ulcers are open sores that can occur in various areas of the body. When ulcers occur in the stomach they are called peptic or gastric ulcers. Approximately 85 percent of stomach ulcers are caused by the bacteria *H. pylori* in the stomach. Many doctors prescribe antibiotics to kill the bacteria, but patients often still have pain associated with the ulcer. To combat the pain, you can try a mixture of 1 teaspoon of apple cider vinegar and ½ teaspoon of baking soda. The mixture may fizz a bit when you first combine it but that is normal. When the fizzing subsides add 8 ounces of water and drink.

14: PROMOTES CANCER PREVENTION

Each and every year, cancer diminishes the quality of countless people's lives and takes the lives of many more. While the underlying causes of many cancerous conditions can't be determined, the evolution and progression of cancer throughout the body's cells, organs, and systems can be tracked easily. Carcinogenic properties and elements come into contact with cells and attack their biological foundation and create a harmful version of the cell that then communicates with other cells within the body, spreading the cancerous infection. These communications can infiltrate the cells, organs, and systems throughout the body, spreading the cancer progressively over time.

Because the countless toxins, carcinogens, and chemicals that we encounter daily contribute to the development of these cancerous takeovers, many people are now searching for all-natural preventative remedies. Surprisingly, baking soda can be used in this health-improving area too. With 1 teaspoon of baking soda dissolved in an 8-ounce glass of water consumed daily, the cells are protected with baking soda's pH-balancing effects. With the reduction of inflammation that also results from the consumption of baking soda, the cells are exposed to far less carcinogenic substances that induce cancerous changes. While improving immunity, protecting against inflammation, and battling the toxic infiltration of cancerous cells into the body's organs and systems, baking soda also ensures the maintenance of health throughout the brain and body naturally by simply maintaining balance.

CAUTIOUS PROMOTIONS OF NATURAL CANCER PREVENTIONS

When the public is presented with the latest news on preventative or curative approaches to cancer, people should be aware that the medical community takes major precautions in their promotion of therapies and medicines, which means that some helpful, effective approaches to treatment get left in the dark due to a lack of Food and Drug Administration (FDA) approval or pharmaceutical backing. Some all-natural therapies may be studied at length and even show promise in preventing or alleviating cancer but may ultimately be "hushed" and not gain mainstream traction. It would behoove anyone concerned with all-natural treatments for cancer to research, read, and interview any source available who may have accurate and up-to-date information that may be left out of the mainstream.

15: ENHANCES EXERCISE REPARATION

Every time you exercise, your body benefits in countless ways: the brain produces hormones to promote health and happiness; the digestive system produces adequate enzymes for optimal absorption and distribution of nutrients; and blood circulation improves not only in support of the body's many systems' functions but also so that oxygen can be more readily available for every cell, organ, and system. With the implementation of exercise, the muscles move through a process of breakdown and rebuilding to become stronger and healthier over a 24–72-hour period following each workout. While the muscles break down and repair, a natural byproduct produced in the breakdown process is lactic acid. While this organic compound is natural and automatically produced during any physical exertion that challenges the muscles, it is the lactic acid lingering in the muscles that causes stiffness, pain, and soreness. For those who would rather avoid this sore side effect following exercise, plentiful products promise to offer relief and minimize the aftereffects of workouts. As with almost every other product available, though, these lactic acid–reducing pills and potions can contain harsh chemicals and additives that not only counter your exercise efforts but can also be harmful to your overall health.

Baking soda can be used to regulate this common issue naturally. With 1 teaspoon of baking soda dissolved in an 8-ounce glass of water, the blood and organs can be rejuvenated and supported with pH-balancing effects that help rid the body of lactic acid naturally. In addition, a paste made of 1 part aloe vera and 2 parts baking soda can be topically applied to the areas stressed during workouts for reducing inflammation and assistance in the reparation process without any chemicals or additives.

THE DANGERS OF POOR REPARATION TECHNIQUES

When starting a new workout routine, one of the most common mistakes is to neglect proper muscle reparation. With lactic acid buildup in the muscles, pain and discomfort can interfere with future workouts and lead to a disinterest in continuing a healthy exercise program. With natural aids such as baking soda that can help regulate pH and improve the body's metabolism of lactic acid, those who engage in exercise can improve their recovery while naturally maximizing their overall health as well.

16: PROMOTES HEALTHY KIDNEY FUNCTION

The kidneys are an important and valuable part of your body's systems. From acting as a filter that purges the body of toxins to promoting healthy hormone production, the kidneys are an essential set of organs that not only protect health but also promote it. With the massive amount of toxic components that the body comes into contact with daily, the liver provides the cells, organs, and systems with a natural filter that helps remove harmful chemicals, synthetic compounds, and excess waste from the entire body. In performing these filtration functions, the kidneys help maintain overall health and wellness.

Knowing that the kidneys help provide protection against illness and disease, many people are taking on the task of minimizing their toxicity by making a conscious effort to reduce their ingestion and exposure to toxic elements, thereby improving the health of the kidneys and related organs and systems. When you eat a clean diet free of foods and beverages riddled with chemicals, preservatives, and additives, your body can absorb and utilize nutrients from your food for your body's maximum benefit.

By adding 1 teaspoon of baking soda dissolved in 1 cup of water to your daily routine, the regulation of your body's pH and the balancing effects for hormones, blood quality, nutrient absorption, and digestion all provide the kidneys with healing and health-promoting benefits. With highly functioning kidneys, baking soda consumers enjoy less toxicity and better health everyday naturally.

BAKING SODA HELPS SLOW THE DECLINE OF KIDNEY FUNCTION TOO

A study at the Royal London Hospital surveyed 139 patients with advanced chronic kidney disease and found that a daily dose of baking soda (in addition to their regular care) helped slow their kidney decline by about two thirds compared to the patients who did not take the baking soda. The patients who took the baking soda also saw an improvement in other areas of nutrition as well.

17: ALLEVIATES SKIN IRRITATIONS FROM CHICKEN POX AND MEASLES

The Center for Disease Control and Prevention (CDC) estimates that more than 20 million people contract the measles or chicken pox worldwide annually. Between these two diseases, countless people suffer from skin irritations such as redness, itchiness, inflammation, and rashes and sores that can create open wounds. The risk of infection from bacteria and toxins in the environment sky-rocket when these conditions develop, increasing the incidence of serious illness or even death. Additionally, with their compromised immune systems, these afflicted patients not only suffer from these skin diseases themselves, but also pose a serious threat to surrounding family members and acquaintances who have not been immunized. While the debate against immunizations and vaccinations is prevalent in developed countries where adequate care is available, many people around the world have little or no access to the health-care that would assist in the prevention or recovery of these diseases. In situations where citizens are contracting and developing the symptoms associated with these two conditions, baking soda can help shorten the duration of the disease and alleviate the intensity of the symptoms.

The application of a baking soda solution created by combining a one-to-one ratio of baking soda and aloe, results in a reduction in redness, irritation, inflammation, and severity of itchiness. By consuming a daily dose of 1 teaspoon of baking soda dissolved in 1 cup of water, patients also experience an improvement in immune system functioning to reduce the effects of the skin conditions on the cells, organs, and systems. Baking soda is one of the most effective treatments for these skin irritations and it acts safely and naturally without the risk of any side effects.

18: CLEANSES MOUTH DEVICES (DENTURES AND RETAINERS)

The conditions that can lead to the need for a mouth device can happen to anyone regardless of age, gender, socioeconomic status, or even their attentiveness to oral care. Whether the device be a retainer or a set of dentures, the need to keep the mouth piece clean is essential. With the existence of bacteria being prominent in the mouth, the care for the teeth, gums, and tongue become more than optional, making proper oral hygiene essential. The risk of infection from contaminated mouth pieces makes the care and cleaning of these devices a serious issue. With bacterial infections being responsible for serious conditions including death, the maintenance of these devices can either promote or compromise health.

Rinsing these oral devices in organic apple cider vinegar causes the microbes, bacteria, and viruses that can wreak havoc on the body to be diminished, depleted, and disrupted in their spreading and ability to invade the body. While apple cider vinegar rinses can be healthy for the fighting of caustic microbes, a paste created from a one-to-one ratio of coconut oil and baking soda can be used to gently scrub the surfaces and crevasses of mouth devices. With no worry of chemical residue, staining, bleaching, or infecting microbes and bacteria, anyone who uses a mouth device can live happily and healthfully with baking soda to thank.

CREATE AN OVERNIGHT SOAK

You can also use baking soda to create an effective overnight soak for dentures and other mouth devices. Simply soak devices in a solution of 2 teaspoons of baking soda dissolved in warm water.

19: ACTS AS AN ANTACID

With countless conditions contributing to the development of gastric acid abnormalities, the health industry has developed multiple products that promise to provide relief from the symptoms associated with the condition. Between bad breath, stomach aches, indigestion, and pain throughout the esophagus, stomach, and bowels, acid reflux issues can wreak havoc on everyday life and overall health. While many patients suffer from acid reflux as a result of medication, heredity, or health issues, even lifestyle habits such as dietary choices, excessive caffeine consumption, or even poor exercise and sleep habits can all interrupt normal gastric acid maintenance. Through the implementation of healthy life choices like limiting fast food, sugar, processed foods that contain additives, sodium, and fat, while exercising regularly, sleeping adequate lengths of time, and restricting medication use to only times that are absolutely necessary many people have seen an improvement in their acid-related pains.

By implementing a baking soda regimen that involves the consumption of ½ teaspoon of baking soda dissolved in ½ cup of water, you can find immediate relief against gastric acid symptoms. The added benefit of this on-the-spot immediate relief concoction is that, unlike over-the-counter medications and antacids, baking soda provides relief without side effects while also promoting the health and healing of the body's cells, organs, and systems that can be adversely affected by gastric acid issues. Because baking soda can regulate your pH, assist in nutrient absorption, and aid in digestion, it can be the best possible alternative for any patient who consumes antacids regularly.

USE IN MODERATION

As with any antacid medication, if you take too much baking soda, you will neutralize the acid in your stomach. This can result in your stomach producing more acid to compensate, causing you to take more baking soda and thus forming a vicious cycle. Remember that baking soda is not a long-term solution to heartburn. You will need to discover the underlying cause of your heartburn in order to find a long-term solution that works for you.

20: RELIEVES CANKER SORES

Canker sores are signs of underlying health issues that often require immediate attention. These shallow sores in the mouth, below the gum lines, or throughout the interior of the mouth should not be confused with the fever blisters that result from Herpes Simplex 1 and require antibiotics. Canker sores can result from a diet rich in spicy, fatty, or nutrient-depleted foods, but can also result from illness, injury, or chronic conditions that cause fluctuations in hormones, pH balance, and even body temperature. With medications that are often purchased or prescribed in an effort to minimize symptoms, shorten duration, or prevent the recurrence of the sore, the patient can fall victim to side effects that actually worsen the condition instead of cure it.

For canker sore sufferers who choose to opt for all-natural alternatives, a combination of two baking soda applications, such as a one-to-one paste of water and baking soda applied to the canker sore for 3–5 minutes before rinsing, as well as a mouth rinse of ½ teaspoon of baking soda and 1 tablespoon of coconut oil to be swished for 10 minutes before spitting and brushing, can be the answers they seek.

Baking soda's abilities to combat bacteria, improve blood flow, maintain pH balance, fight acidity, and regulate hormones combine to help the body rid itself of the underlying condition, improve the immune system, and provide protective prevention against future development of canker sores. If the sore results from injury, the open wound is also protected by baking soda's preventative measures against infection. Ensuring safe healing, baking soda makes canker sore suffering a thing of the past...safely and naturally.

THE BENEFITS OF COCONUT OIL

While the mouth-rinsing process involving coconut oil has been long used by countless individuals for many years, few people are aware of its immense benefits. By swishing the coconut oil in the mouth for 10–20 minutes daily, the healthy balance of good bacteria is preserved while the harmful germs and microbes are eliminated naturally...with the added benefit of whiter teeth.

21: REDUCES BLOATING

There are a number of marketing ploys that poke fun at bloating: Thanksgiving dinners that make it impossible to button pants while watching the celebratory football game, a side of broccoli that suddenly makes a lunch meeting embarrassing, and so on, but bloating is a serious matter that is indicative of the digestive system being overwhelmed and unable to digest foods properly.

Excessive gas production in the digestive tract can lead to the condition commonly referred to as "bloating." While there are a number of situations including overeating, dehydration, medications, and a variety of medical conditions (even pregnancy) that can lead to this uncomfortable condition, the plentiful array of medications and treatments available for the minimizing of gas production and buildup can actually worsen the condition or cause other disruptive side effects such as diarrhea, belching, dizziness, fatigue, and so on.

By choosing to integrate a number of health-improving habits such as increasing water consumption, avoiding carbonation, increasing the consumption of greens and leafy vegetables while avoiding cruciferous vegetables (broccoli, cauliflower, and Brussels sprouts), and maintaining a diet that includes smaller-sized meals every 3 hours as opposed to one, two, or three large meals, the body can avoid the stimulations and situations that make bloating almost inevitable.

Baking soda can play a natural role in minimizing bloating by moving through the digestive tract with its pH-balancing effects. Returning the pH to neutral levels, the body's gasses can be calmed and the digestive processes, acids, and enzymes can return to their natural state and foods can be broken down normally without issues and disruptions. One teaspoon of baking soda dissolved in a 4–6-ounce glass of water can help alleviate the issues associated with bloating quickly and naturally. So the next time you feel bloated, forego the processed products and opt for a simple solution with baking soda instead.

22: CALMS UNEASY STOMACHS

Stress, depression, sudden triggers and surprising situations, food aversions, and medical conditions are just a few of the most common contributors to the onset of uneasy and upset stomachs. Whether the condition lasts for only a few minutes to an hour, or extends and intensifies throughout the night, uneasy stomachs can feel torturous and even excruciating when the queasiness fails to subside. In severe cases of uneasy stomachs turning to intense medical symptoms of a more serious medical condition, a physician should be consulted immediately. For the average case of uneasiness, though, there are a number of natural remedies that can be utilized for treating the uneasiness, shortening its duration, and preventing its progression. With natural healing applications such as ingestion of small amounts of gingerroot, consumption of stomach soothing teas such as chamomile, and breathing exercises that ensure delivery of oxygen to the brain and body, the brain and body can regulate the digestive system's natural processes without interference.

Baking soda enters into the treatment process of uneasy stomachs by targeting the stomach and the brain.

Hormonal imbalances that can stimulate or inhibit the production and excretion of essential hormones (especially those in "fight or flight" that can cause the blood to leave the stomach due to the sudden onset of stress), can be fixed with baking soda's ability to restore a balance in the blood and brain. In addition, 1 teaspoon of baking soda consumed in an 8-ounce glass of water can help aid in the digestion of undigested food particles while aiding the digestive enzymes and acids that can all be disrupted in uneasiness. By combining these natural treatment options, the average uneasy stomach can be resolved quickly, while restoring the essential balance to the body and brain for optimal health and functioning.

23: EASES ALLERGIES

Every year, millions of people develop allergies to foods, toxins, and irritants in the foods and environments that they encounter. With these allergic reactions, the symptoms range from mild such as watery eyes and runny noses to severe such as inflammatory responses that can lead to serious anaphylactic shock. While the more severe allergies can result in hospitalization after exposure, the milder type of allergies are more common. Pharmaceutical companies create countless varieties of allergy medications that are designed to treat the stuffiness, irritated eyes, sinus pressure, and coughs that are commonly associated with daily or seasonal allergies. While these medications (prescription and over-the-counter) can provide relief, the most commonly reported side effects are those that adversely affect energy levels, cognitive functioning, and heart rate.

By using all-natural remedies such as baking soda, allergy sufferers can safely treat their allergic reactions while also initiating preventative protection that can alleviate or relieve allergy intensity and frequency. By combining 1 teaspoon of baking soda in a 4–6-ounce glass of green tea and consuming it at the beginning of your day, you can provide your body with potent anti-inflammatory agents that combine to prevent the incidence of inflammation throughout the sinuses, the airways, and even the body's cells. In fighting inflammatory responses, the allergies' underlying causes can be combatted with natural inhibitory effects. In addition to fighting inflammation, baking soda can also improve your body's pH level to ensure that the bloodstream is able to combat microbes and illnesses while also encouraging the health of the liver and kidneys for optimal purging of toxins from the body.

WHEN THE LIVER IS JEOPARDIZED

With the liver helping the body detoxify, this organ plays an integral role in optimizing and maintaining health. When jeopardized, the effects can include exhaustion, mental fogginess, and an onset of illness and disease. By assisting the liver with a clean diet and all-natural ingredients (such as pH-balancing baking soda), the detoxification process is less grueling for the ever-important liver, allowing it to maximize its efforts at natural detoxification successfully.

24: TREATS YEAST INFECTIONS

Due to the over-development of yeast, a yeast infection can take over the beneficial bacteria that usually help maintain the health of the parts and processes involved in the reproductive system. Usually these helpful bacteria help maintain a healthy pH in the body—the delicate balance that helps ensure that odors, discharge, and the daily activities of everyday life are unable to interfere with the moisture-related issues that can contribute to yeast overgrowth. But when there is an overgrowth of negative bacteria it overwhelms the helpful bacteria and they become compromised.

While the symptoms of yeast infections such as foul odor, painful burning, intense itchiness, and an abundant discharge can all be uncomfortable, the underlying issues are the true concern. With millions of men and women experiencing yeast infections each year, pharmaceutical companies and female hygiene product manufacturers have developed a dizzying number of wipes, lotions, lubricants, pills, and potions that promise to relieve the symptoms while also counteracting the underlying issues. While these products and medications seem promising, they can be very unsafe and lead to an exacerbation of the initial cause.

Baking soda can be used in a number of applications that can help the internal balance of pH, and return the body's hormonal levels to normal. All of these benefits result from the consumption of 1 teaspoon of baking soda dissolved in an 8-ounce glass of water every 4 hours after the onset of a yeast infection. In addition to the consumption of baking soda, a cleansing rinse of the same solution can be used as a rinse during the shower to help return pH balances to normal. Safely and naturally, baking soda can be the perfect treatment—inside and out—for yeast infection sufferers.

QUESTIONABLE INGREDIENTS AND SERIOUS CONSEQUENCES

A growing percentage of the population is paying attention to the chemicals and additives that are being introduced to their bodies. Feminine hygiene products can be unassuming purchases that release countless questionable ingredients into the body with effects that are still yet to be determined. By opting for all-natural, organic products and treatments, anyone concerned with long-term health can safeguard themselves against inadvertent exposure effectively.

25: REHYDRATES YOUR BODY

Adequate hydration in the body assists and supports far more functions than most people recognize. From the smallest cell membranes to the largest organs, hydration is directly responsible for ensuring that maintenance and stability is upheld. Without proper hydration, the cells, organs, and systems not only diminish in their own right, but also begin to deteriorate the functioning of the cells, organs, and systems that rely on them. With the onset of dehydration, a domino-like effect begins to wreak havoc on the body with serious consequences occurring in the very elements that effect overall health and well-being. Chronic conditions, even cancers, can take hold of compromised cells that lack the impenetrable protection that comes with hydration and hydro-support.

With the implementation of a water-consumption regimen that involves a minimum of 8 (8-ounce) glasses of water daily, the body can receive the minimum recommended water requirement. Any vigorous exercise or environmental condition that results in excessive sweating will increase this amount, obviously, but the minimum 8 cups (64 ounces) should remain the focus of anyone working to improve their hydration. Baking soda helps improve the body's ability to retain hydration by maintaining the body's natural pH, improving the digestive system's ability to absorb nutrients essential in the hydration process, and maintain proper blood flow to ensure those nutrients are able to be utilized by the cells, organs, and systems that rely on vitamins, minerals, and antioxidants for proper functioning. The simple addition of ½ teaspoon of baking soda in just one or two of your 8-ounce daily glasses of water can help ensure adequate hydration throughout the day and night naturally.

THIRST AS AN INDICATION OF DEHYDRATION

Most people wait until they feel thirsty to rehydrate, but few realize that thirst is an indication that dehydration has already set in. When thirstiness occurs, the body's cells, organs, and systems are already suffering from the depletion of essential water that helps the functions and processes that they are each responsible for. Drinking an 8-ounce glass of water each hour, and more when exercising, can help ensure adequate hydration throughout the day.

26: KILLS FUNGI, MILDEW, AND MOLD

With the growth of mold, mildew, and fungi running rampant in hot, dark, damp, humid places, many consumers seek products that can prevent, combat, or kill these growths that adversely affect the health of plants, people, and environments. Because of the slow spread of the spores of these multicellular filaments scientifically referred to as "hyphae," any area can be invaded over time. The spread of these natural spores can be a slow progression over time that is almost unnoticeable to the human eye, but the intensity of this harmful spread can be catastrophic. The spores that help the spread of mold, mildew, and fungi can be inhaled into the lungs of humans and wreak havoc on the body's systems. Starting in the respiratory system, these spores can inhibit the transport of oxygen, increase inflammation in the airways and throughout the sinuses, and infect the bloodstream and organs. With such intense consequences, there's no question that these potentially harmful growths need to be contained to natural areas that do not adversely affect people.

While widespread overgrowths of mold, mildew, and fungi may require professional removal of structures such as drywall to ensure safety precautions are in place, the milder spreads of these natural spores can be treated with an application of a simple solution made of water and baking soda. With this 1-part–baking soda to 2-parts-water solution poured into a spray bottle, anyone can apply the natural alternative to chemical laden mold, mildew, and fungi removers. Safe for use on home surfaces as well as plants, this solution is a simple and inexpensive treatment that will keep you and your loved ones healthy and happy without the concern of the potentially harmful spores.

27: COMBATS AND TREATS PARASITES

Parasites can infiltrate the body in a number of ways, each one resorting to a different mode of leeching the life (literally) out of a human host. In all cases, the parasite involved seeks to achieve one goal: to forage the host for sustenance that can provide the necessary nourishment to survive and thrive. The scope and severity of parasitic infection symptoms are dependent upon the type of parasite and the area in which the infection occurs. The heart, lungs, brain, liver, kidney, digestive tract, and eyes are the most common areas that parasites thrive because these organs can provide enough nutrients for a parasite to live. If these areas and organs fall victim to a parasitic infection, it can lead to serious complications, illness, disease, and even death.

Through ingestion of infected food or liquids or exposure to parasitic environments, the human body can be riddled with leeching parasites that cause dizziness, vomiting, diarrhea, pneumonia, migraines, and heart failure. With this in mind, the medications that are commonly provided in treatment programs for parasites can be equally catastrophic in their effects on the body, ironically posing the same potential side effects as the parasitic symptoms.

In an effort to prevent the invasion of parasites or combat the spread of an existing parasitic infestation, medical professionals have witnessed natural relief when infected patients simply consume a solution of 1 tablespoon of baking soda and 1 cup of water up to four times daily for 3 days. Not only does the baking soda combat acidity in the bloodstream and organs, but the effects on the digestive system help purge the parasite from the body naturally. While many doctors may still urge a patient to continue a more medicalized approach to ridding the body of parasites, the all-natural baking soda alterative has been used in countries around the world with great success for countless years.

28: EASES COUGHS

Whether your cough is an everyday occurrence that accompanies your allergies or a more serious symptom of a respiratory issue, there are a number of over-the-counter and prescription medications that promise to provide relief. While these lozenges, syrups, pills, and potions may seem enticing when you only seek peace from persistent, disruptive coughs, the ingredients and additives in these applications can be questionable. Packed with synthetic substances that may be unnecessary for your condition and may even pose a threat to your health by complicating other existing conditions, these seemingly harmless treatment options may not be the right choice for you.

The constant tickle in your throat that creates the urge to cough can also make your body endure muscle spasms and tightening, making muscle pain and weakness another undesirable symptom of persistent coughing. For an all-natural approach to resolving the underlying issue of coughing, preventing the urge to cough, and even aiding in the repair of the adverse effects a severe cough can have on the muscles, patients need look no further than a few simple ingredients that are most likely already in their kitchens.

Baking soda has the ability to reduce inflammation, and the tickle at the back of your throat can be alleviated with a simple solution of 1 teaspoon of baking soda dissolved in an 8-ounce glass of water in the morning. This solution also helps combat lactic acid buildup in muscles, relieving soreness and tension naturally. Additionally, consuming 1 tablespoon of organic apple cider vinegar in an 8-ounce glass of water daily will rid the body of bacteria, viruses, fungi, and microbes that can contribute to the development of respiratory illnesses. Simply and easily these two approaches combine to relieve a cough with the safety and security that can only be found in nature.

29: SOOTHES SORE THROATS

A sore throat can start any time, any day, and for any number of reasons. The most common sore throats stem from an infection triggered by bacteria, viruses, or microbes and can signal the onset of a more pervasive illness. When the immune system is healthy, a sore throat can be treated quickly and easily with the use of all-natural remedies that can restore and support the body's healthy functions. While it can be tempting to either ignore a sore throat or treat it with a myriad of tinctures, pills, and sprays, the pharmaceutical varieties of sore throat remedies can exacerbate the underlying issue or leave your sore throat feeling relieved but the underlying condition unresolved.

When working to combat a sore throat at its source, your treatment plan should include a topical pain reliever that alleviates inflammation and a strategic internal approach that will help rid the body of bacteria, viruses, and microbes while boosting the immune system.

Baking soda has a natural alkalizing ability, which means it can neutralize the acidic pH of the body that encourages infectious illnesses and diseases to thrive. With a simple throat spray consisting of 1 tablespoon of baking soda and 4 tablespoons of water, a soothing spritz of baking soda into the back of the mouth can provide immediate relief of inflammation, irritation, redness, and pain while also combatting bacteria on the spot. Consuming a combination of 1 teaspoon of baking soda and ½ cup of water can improve the blood's quality, fight bacterial infection internally, and fend off toxicity that all contribute to sore throats. The implementation of a high vitamin C regimen, as well as 1 tablespoon of apple cider vinegar diluted in ½ cup of water daily can also help fight viruses, microbes, and fungal infections safely and naturally.

30: MINIMIZES THE LENGTH OF COLDS AND THE FLU

Suffering from the common cold or the seasonal flu can be devastating to the body, mind, and spirit. Between the muscle soreness and stiffness, aching head, lack of energy, and inability to focus, the symptoms of these common illnesses can really upset everyday life. With new strains of these illnesses popping up each year, vaccines and preventative medicines that were previously effective now fail to deliver on the promise of protection against these invasive infections and their uncomfortable symptoms. More serious cases of these illnesses can be particularly difficult to combat, and the longer they persist in patients, the greater their risk of succumbing to pneumonia and even death. And when it comes to the side effects of common medications prescribed for these illnesses, they can be even more detrimental than the original threat posed by the cold and flu—especially for pregnant women and their fetuses.

Doubting the effectiveness and safety of the typical preventative measures and treatment options commonly prescribed, many cold and flu sufferers have turned to all-natural methods of prevention and restorative health options. Of the many tried-and-true alternatives available, one of the most effective is baking soda.

With the ability to restore the body's natural balance of pH, hormones, and blood health, baking soda is able to sweep through the body and cleanse the cells, organs, and systems of harmful bacteria and toxins. Baking soda also helps support the digestive system, liver, and kidneys in purging the unhealthy microbes that can extend the duration of illnesses. One teaspoon of baking soda dissolved in ½ cup of water can be consumed every 2 hours for internal assistance with combatting these illnesses. The same solution can be used in a neti pot to help purge mucus and microbes from the sinus cavities where sickness can linger and foster further infection.

31: BALANCES pH

The pH of your blood plays an important role in your body's essential processes, yet it can be dumbfounding to realize how few people take their pH into account when evaluating their health. A normal pH is 7.4. If your pH is lower than 7.4 your blood is acidic; if your pH is higher than 7.4 your blood is alkaline. Acidic or alkaline blood can interfere with processes in the body and can be a result of disease. Your primary care physician can test your blood to determine the pH of your blood.

The most amazing part of trying to achieve optimal wellness can be learning about the inner workings of the body and how each choice we make throughout the day can either move us toward our health goals or set us back. We know healthy diet, exercise, and lifestyle choices all contribute (or detract) from the body's health and well-being, but there are less obvious, seemingly minute considerations that can also have enormous benefits or consequences to our health.

For the support and maintenance of your essential body processes, a balanced pH is crucial. An optimal pH balance not only helps break down foods, ensure proper digestion, streamline the delivery of nutrients throughout the body, and restore muscle support from properly processed proteins and carbohydrates, but it also helps each of the cells that support these processes efficiently perform their intended functions. To help balance your body's pH, you should avoid consuming too much meat, dairy, processed food, and acidic liquid. Also be sure to add strength and endurance exercises to your routine.

The alkaline stability of baking soda is able to optimize the pH balance of the entire body. Completely void of adverse side effects, 1 teaspoon of baking soda can be dissolved in ½ cup of water and consumed daily. So while a clean diet, invigorating exercise routine, and healthy lifestyle choices will all help bring individuals closer to optimal health, the addition of baking soda and its pH-balancing effects can (and will!) maximize those efforts.

32: RELIEVES GOUT

Gout sufferers must endure the shooting pain, aching, and stiffness that results from the onset of this unpleasant condition. Between morning pains that keep toes and fingers from moving freely to an intensified painfulness that accompanies poor dietary choices, the symptoms and effects of gout can adversely affect an individual's quality of life. Gout involves a uric acid buildup. Excess uric acid moves into joints and hardens into crystallized masses. When this hardening occurs, the pain, stiffness, and aching become a daily burden and can be exacerbated by consuming meals that are high in fat and sugar or contain certain seafood.

While many medical professionals claim that prescription medications are the key to recovery, the truth is that all-natural approaches to minimizing gout and its symptoms are available to anyone who has access to a few simple, inexpensive, and easy-to-obtain products...baking soda being one of the most effective.

Baking soda is heralded for its ability to regulate pH, which means that it can break down uric acid in the bloodstream and promote the liver's ability to process the excess acid while also supporting the kidneys in ridding it from the body. In addition to 1 teaspoon of baking soda in a 4-ounce glass of water consumed daily, 1 teaspoon of virgin coconut oil consumed daily has been shown to reduce inflammation in the joints. Apple cider vinegar has also been shown to improve gout by cleansing the bloodstream of toxic substances and organic compounds, such as those produced from excessive uric acid production.

THE UNKNOWN PAINS ASSOCIATED WITH GOUT

While gout is a common disease that affects a growing percentage of the population around the world each year, it's surprising to learn that the foot pain that often strikes gout sufferers can go undiagnosed as a symptom of gout if it is not brought to the attention of a physician. Gout pain that radiates from the toes can lead to serious discomfort, stiffness, disfigurement, as well as serious interference in everyday life activities. This is why foot pain should be mentioned to a physician whenever it continues for a week or longer. Changes in diet and lifestyle, as well as the implementation of natural healing ingredients (like baking soda) can all help alleviate this pain naturally.

33: TREATS UTIs

Urinary tract infections (also known as UTIs) are infections that inhibit the flow of urine through the urethra. This condition, while common, is a serious one that can cause severe damage to the body and its essential systems. Urinary tract infections specifically affect the urinary tract and urethra, usually due to a bacterial infection that impedes the normal flow of urine, increases the pH of the blood and urine in the bladder and kidneys, and causes bacteria and microbes to adhere to the walls of the ureters and urethra. When this infection takes hold, the symptoms can be excruciating and include the frequent urge to urinate, a burning sensation that accompanies urination, and eventual pain in the lower back. Uncomfortable to say the least, each of these symptoms signifies a serious dysfunction taking place in one or more of the body's organs and systems.

With the use of baking soda, the kidneys receive pH-balancing regulation that helps detoxify the blood and urine of impurities and other harmful substances that can impede the natural flow of urine through the urinary tract. The bacteria sticking to the walls of the urethra are also purged through the antibacterial effects of baking soda, allowing for even more immediate relief of the underlying issue. Baking soda also helps prevent the spread of bacteria to the kidneys, which could otherwise result in serious damage.

To naturally fight UTIs, simply drink 1 teaspoon of baking soda dissolved in a 2-ounce glass of all-natural cranberry juice every 2 hours. The ingestion of the baking soda helps return your body to a healthy pH while cranberry juice has been proven to improve urinary tract health.

34: MINIMIZES MIGRAINES

Migraine sufferers seek help billions of times throughout the world each year. Serious symptoms can include sharp, pulsating pains that coincide with exposure to sounds and light and chronic throbbing pains that only subside after retreating from sounds and light. Migraines are intrusive and painful conditions. While the medical community has identified certain areas of the brain in migraine-sufferers that seem to be overly sensitive to light and sound when they become over-stimulated, the underlying causes of migraines and the factors that make certain individuals more susceptible to migraine onset are still unknown.

In an effort to calm these physiological reactions to stimulants in the body and the environment, many migraine sufferers find themselves searching for relief in a prescription or over-the-counter medication. While extreme cases of headaches might warrant in-depth analysis to rule out other serious conditions that can produce migraines, most migraine sufferers can reap the benefits of baking soda for all-natural relief.

With 1 teaspoon of baking soda dissolved in an 8-ounce glass of water, migraines can be minimized or resolved completely. By targeting the pH balance of the blood and the brain, this simple baking soda solution can help restore a positive balance to the blood, organs, and systems to help alleviate the pressures and imbalances that can contribute to migraines. With the added benefit of baking soda's ability to restore a healthy balance to hormones and brain chemistry, the consumption of baking soda can help relieve migraines when they strike while also preventing migraines in the future.

TRY A BAKING SODA BATH

Although it may not help with all types of migraines, some sufferers have said that a relaxing bath with baking soda in the water helps with their migraine pain. The baking soda in the bath water helps your body detox and can restore balance to your body's systems. Try incorporating a baking soda bath into your daily migraine management and see if it can make a difference for you too.

35: HELPS HEADACHES

Countless headache sufferers turn to multiple varieties of treatments that promise to provide relief from the life-altering pain that can strike at any time. Whether it's due to an injury, upset in brain chemical balance, or a simple biochemical reaction to something in the environment, a headache can strike at any time. When a headache occurs it can be tempting to turn to readily marketed pharmaceuticals that promise to ease the pain, but the adverse effects to the body's cells, organs, and systems can lead to the development of chronic illnesses and diseases that extend far beyond headaches.

When a headache strikes, it can derail every aspect of your day. Between affecting your demeanor to interrupting your focus, headaches can make even the simplest parts of your day more difficult. With the addition of natural, holistic approaches, headaches can be relieved *and* prevented. If a headache suddenly strikes, lemon-infused water containing baking soda is the perfect cure. Totally lacking in side effects, this effective solution is the best for headaches, helping to relieve dehydration, hormonal abnormalities, and even toxicity. By boosting immunity, strengthening liver and kidney functioning, and ensuring optimal brain chemistry, lemon's rich sources of vitamin C and potent antioxidants combine with baking soda for a healthy headache-relieving elixir.

This simple combination of natural ingredients can be made quickly and easily, providing almost immediate relief with every sip while also supporting the health and well-being of the entire body.

WHEN YOU EXPERIENCE A HEADACHE, SIMPLY CREATE THE FOLLOWING ELIXIR:

16 cups water
Juice of 4 medium lemons
½ cup baking soda

Combine all ingredients in a large pitcher and stir to dissolve.

This solution can be stored in an airtight pitcher in the refrigerator for up to 7 days.

RECOMMENDATIONS FOR USE:

Consume as often as necessary (optimally, about 1 cup per hour) until the headache subsides.

36: SOOTHES SORE TEETH AND GUMS

Mouth pain can be one of the most aggravating forms of physical pain. Toothaches, tingling, sensitivity to hot and cold, gum recession, and gum inflammation can all leave a patient with mild irritation or pain so severe that it distracts and detracts from the enjoyment of everyday life. When you consider the extent to which the mouth is used, it can be easy to understand how everyday activities such as eating, drinking, and even breathing can all be adversely affected by mouth pain. In an effort to prevent the conditions that contribute to mouth pain, dentists belonging to the American Dental Association recommend brushing and flossing at least twice daily and incorporating a mouth rinse to help rid the mouth of bacteria and microbes that can hide in the crevices a toothbrush and floss don't come into contact with. While a number of products are available for oral hygiene and the relief of mouth pain, these products can contain harsh chemicals and additives that may be counterproductive in the pursuit of optimal, pain-free dental health.

Baking soda can be used as an all-natural alternative to store-bought dental applications, providing anti-bacterial, anti-inflammatory, and immunity-boosting benefits that not only protect mouth health but also promote and safeguard the health of the entire body. By maintaining the health of the mouth, the body is protected against harmful microbes that can be swallowed and distributed throughout the body, wreaking havoc on the cells, organs, and systems. A paste consisting of 1 tablespoon of baking soda and 1 tablespoon of water can be safely used to clean the teeth and other surfaces of the mouth as often as necessary. To make an accompanying mouth rinse, combine 1 tablespoon of coconut oil and 1 teaspoon of baking soda and swish the solution for 10–20 minutes to extract germs and bacteria that can lead to the conditions that cause mouth pain.

37: MAKES A pH-BALANCING BLUEBERRY SMOOTHIE

The positive effects of an optimized pH are astounding. Helping to improve everything from blood health to hormonal balance, digestion to muscle maintenance, the proper pH ensures that acids in the body can be controlled and maintained for peak performance at all times. Even cognitive functioning, immunity, and protection against serious illnesses such as cancer can be rooted in the optimization of pH balance.

While 1 teaspoon of baking soda dissolved in an 8-ounce glass of water can help restore and regulate the body's pH, there are other surprising ways to consume servings of baking soda that can contribute to the health and well-being of the body's cells, organs, and systems. One of the easiest (and tastiest!) ways to consume your daily pH-balancing dose of baking soda is to whip up this delicious blueberry smoothie. With ingredients that include potassium-rich bananas, iron-packed spinach, and sweet almond milk, this smoothie only needs a sprinkle of 2 teaspoons of baking soda to provide two people with a pH-healing remedy that satisfies the body's needs while satisfying the taste buds too.

TO MAKE THIS DELICIOUS SMOOTHIE, FOLLOW THESE STEPS:

1 cup fresh blueberries
1 medium banana, peeled and frozen
½ cup fresh spinach leaves
3 cups vanilla almond milk
2 teaspoons baking soda
½ cup ice

In a large blender, combine blueberries, banana, spinach, and milk.

Blend on high until all ingredients are thoroughly combined, about 2 minutes.

Sprinkle baking soda into blender while blending, adding ice gradually until desired consistency is achieved.

CANCER-FIGHTING BERRIES

Rich in potent phytochemicals called "anthocyanins," blueberries and blackberries contribute massive amounts of antioxidants that travel through the bloodstream and combat the cancerous changes that can result from free-radical damage. By incorporating these fruits into your daily diet, along with pH-balancing baking soda, you can improve your blood health and protect your body's vital components from cancerous mutations.

38: REMOVES BITTERNESS FROM TEA

There's something so right about a soothing hot cup of tea. With a wide variety of organic, preservative-free, additive-free, non-GMO options gracing the aisles of every grocery store, consumers have lots of convenient and healthy options to choose from. Whether your preference is green, black, white, or chamomile, a cup of tea can be the perfect prescription to calm the nerves, invigorate the system, or bring clarity to an unfocused mind. While tea can be a comforting accompaniment to your day, bitterness can ruin the experience in just a sip. The bad experience of bitter tea can be banned quickly and naturally with the use of baking soda.

In an effort to combat the sour tea taste that can be inherently present in many varieties of store-bought teas, consumers have used sugars, creams, and dairy-free flavorings to mask the bitterness. However, the addition of these products inadvertently transforms their healthy tea into an unhealthy cup of sugar, preservatives, and additives that can contribute serious harm to their overall health.

With a simple sprinkling of ¼ teaspoon of baking soda in a 6-ounce cup of tea, the bitterness of the tea can be resolved naturally. Immediately combatting the acidic tannins that give teas their bitter tastes, baking soda provides a natural pH-balancing solution that helps eliminate bitterness while maintaining the taste of the tea. The baking soda also helps boost the tea's natural health benefits by promoting optimal functioning of the circulatory, nervous, and digestive systems. So the next time you try your cup of tea and are disappointed by its bitter taste, don't let it ruin your mood. You can simply reach for your box of baking soda and sprinkle the health-transforming, bitterness-alleviating remedy right into your cup.

39: TENDERIZES MEAT

With its alkalinity and ability to be dissolved into a simple solution of water or juice, baking soda can be used as a kitchen staple in food preparation, not just odor elimination. In fact, baking soda is one of the easiest all-natural ways to tenderize meat. As the use of marinades has become ever more popular, the average consumer has become increasingly aware of harsh and unhealthy additives in commercial marinades that can harm health. Baking soda has grown in popularity as an inexpensive way to marinate and tenderize meat naturally.

Using baking soda to tenderize less expensive cuts of meat that are traditionally tougher is an economical way to prepare tender slices of beef, pork, or chicken that only takes 15 minutes and costs next to nothing. Anyone who is worried about saving money at the expense of flavor and texture can find reassurance in the use of the baking soda—a surprisingly inexpensive, all-natural approach to making any meat "melt-in-your-mouth" tender.

Mix together a one-to-four ratio of baking soda and water, place the cut of meat in a bowl, and add the baking soda solution until the meat is completely covered. To infuse flavors, create your own marinade by adding spices or juices to the tenderizing solution. Remove the meat from the baking soda solution after it has soaked for about 15–20 minutes. Without rinsing the meat, cook it as directed by your recipe and prepare to enjoy an amazing piece of meat that makes other expensive alternatives seem outrageously overrated.

40: REDUCES THE ACIDITY OF ORANGE JUICE

Orange juice is one of the most widely consumed breakfast foods across the country. Packed with valuable servings of vitamin C and an assortment of vitamins and minerals that help improve immunity, maximize energy levels, and maintain mental clarity, orange juice has long been a breakfast go-to for millions of people who hope to help extend and improve their quality of life. Unfortunately, many people start their day with a pep in their step from the natural sugars of orange juice only to find themselves fighting reflux later. With every sip of this acidic citrus drink, its sweet elixir can transform the pH balance of the gut and the body, resulting in upsets that can affect both body and mind. The feeling of burning sensations in the gut, disruptions in the esophagus, and even dizziness from sugar-crashes can all result from the disruption this seemingly innocent drink can have on the body's natural functions. When the body's pH balance is compromised, the effects can be catastrophic. Adverse effects can impact the digestive system, endocrine system, hormonal balance, and mental stability.

While orange juice may seem like the perfect beverage for your morning breakfast, its high citric acid content can be overwhelming to the body's pH. Luckily, a simple ½ teaspoon of baking soda sprinkled into a 6–8-ounce glass of orange juice can help combat the adverse effects of its acidity. Baking soda is a simple, inexpensive, all-natural option for orange juice lovers who want to continue consuming their favorite vitamin C–rich breakfast accompaniment while still helping their bodies maintain a healthy pH balance.

WATCH OUT FOR THE FIZZ!

When you add an alkaline substance like baking soda to an acid like orange juice you may notice a fizzing reaction. Just stir your orange juice with a straw or spoon and the fizz should dissipate.

41: PREVENTS CURDLING IN MILK

Many sauce recipes or recipes with a cream base call for the addition of milk. While these recipes can develop into delicious sides and sauces for breakfasts, lunches, dinners, salads, soups, and sides, the process of incorporating milk-based ingredients can lead to disastrous outcomes that are far from the ideal. When introduced to heat, or combined with acidic ingredients (wines or citrus juices, for example), milk-based ingredients can curdle and separate, ruining the dish. Taking care in your preparation of hot dishes that contain milk as a main ingredient can ensure that your results come out picture-perfect each and every time.

Baking soda is one solution to combatting acidic reactions that can curdle milk-based concoctions. One teaspoon of baking soda sprinkled and stirred into a pot or pan of your culinary creation's liquids before heating will allow you to combine milk or milk-based products with acidic ingredients without the usual tumultuous turnouts. Baking soda not only helps maintain the integrity of your dish, sauce, or side, but it also ensures that the creation is free of microbes, bacteria, and other questionable health assailants.

WHY DOES MILK CURDLE?

Milk is basically an emulsion of butterfat, protein, and water. When you boil or cook milk over high heat, the emulsion breaks and the milk proteins coagulate and separate from the water, producing curdled milk. The curdled milk does look unappetizing, but it is technically safe to consume.

42: MAKES A STOMACH-SOOTHING GREEN SMOOTHIE

When an upset stomach strikes, the average person either suffers through hours of anguish or turns to over-the-counter medications that promise to provide relief. For those who choose to push through the pain and wait for natural relief, the interruption to daily activities, lapse in sharp mental focus and cognitive functions, and unexpected digestive disruptions can all wreak havoc on a normal daily routine or prevent a restful night's sleep.

The most concerning issue relating to upset stomachs is the cause; whether it be stress, an acidic or spicy ingredient in the diet, or a chronic condition, addressing the body's cause of an upset stomach is not only crucial in calming the upset at the time, but also preventing upsets in the future. Because so few people understand the importance of the body's pH balance, it is completely understandable that most people who suffer from stomach upset turn to the readily available medications that promise to provide relief. For those who resort to medications for relief, the options available can contain questionable ingredients that may exacerbate the underlying condition that led to the development of tummy troubles.

Baking soda adds an alkalizing benefit to this smoothie recipe and helps restore the optimal pH balance that promotes digestive health, toxin removal, and micronutrient absorption and distribution. Adding this simple ingredient to a deliciously sweet spinach smoothie provides the body with maximum nutrition and stomach ache relief at any time of the day or night. This satisfying green smoothie contains all-natural ingredients and a soothing helping of baking soda to tame the average upset stomach quickly, easily, and tastefully.

TO MAKE THIS SMOOTHIE, FOLLOW THESE STEPS:

2 cups fresh spinach
1 medium banana, peeled and frozen
3 cups apple juice
2 teaspoons baking soda

In a large blender, combine all ingredients. Blend on high until all ingredients are fully macerated.

Pour smoothie into two glasses and serve immediately.

43: MAKES AN ANTACID-ALTERNATIVE BANANA SMOOTHIE

Chronic acid reflux sufferers know that few conditions compare to the pain and discomfort that comes with heartburn and indigestion. Burning, coughing, and upset stomachs can be triggered by seemingly any drink or meal, and these acid indigestion symptoms can ruin any day or night. With symptoms lasting for hours or even days, the average acid reflux patient finds themselves desperate for relief in any form, turning to pills, potions, and prescriptions that promise to provide relief. The symptoms of acid reflux can not only be physically discomforting, but they can also contribute to the development of chronic conditions such as ulcers, irritable bowel syndrome (IBS), irritable bowel disease (IBD), or even esophageal irritations. With a soothing smoothie that contains all-natural ingredients that each contribute to digestive health and healing, acid reflux sufferers can find relief in every cup of this banana smoothie recipe.

Baking soda is combined with popular super foods in this recipe for a nutrient-rich smoothie that also provides pH-balancing effects for antacid-like relief throughout the entire digestive system. The anti-inflammatory benefit of baking soda calms irritation, and just 1 teaspoon transforms this simple smoothie into a super smoothie. Also infused with potassium-rich bananas that aid in mineral absorption for optimal digestion, quercetin-packed apples that contribute to the healing of digestive disruption-related conditions (such as ulcers), and antioxidant-abundant cinnamon and cloves for an immune system boost, this simple smoothie packs in some major superfoods.

TO MAKE THIS ALL-NATURAL ANTACID-ALTERNATIVE SMOOTHIE, FOLLOW THESE STEPS:

2 medium bananas, peeled and frozen
1 medium green apple, cored and chopped
1 teaspoon baking soda
1 teaspoon cinnamon
¼ teaspoon cloves
3 cups vanilla almond milk

In a large blender, combine all the ingredients.

Blend on high until all ingredients are fully macerated and thoroughly combined. Pour into two glasses and serve immediately.

44: CREATES A CLEANSING KALE SALAD

With nutrients like iron, potassium, magnesium, B vitamins, vitamin A, vitamin K, and vitamin E, along with potent antioxidants, this perfectly designed salad makes clean eating for cleansing simple *and* satisfying. Pairing deep greens with delicious fruits and nuts, this cleansing kale salad makes for a filling vegetarian meal or snack that provides the body and brain with all of the essentials while satisfying the stomach and the taste buds. With the added benefit of baking soda that contributes pH-balancing benefits and anti-inflammatory agents, the process of "cleansing" that so many find uncomfortable or undesirable can be incorporated into anyone's daily diet with ease.

Helping to remove toxins from the bloodstream, balance the pH of the body's cells and organs, and restore optimal performance of the digestive system, this cleansing kale salad is the all-natural alternative to colon-cleansing medications and over-the-counter options that can lead to extreme cases of diarrhea, bloating, and nausea. Choosing to cleanse with this balanced meal of nutrient-dense foods that nourish the entire body can help anyone optimize their own health and benefit from baking soda's health-restoring properties.

TO MAKE THIS POWER-PACKED SALAD, FOLLOW THESE STEPS:

½ cup extra-virgin olive oil

2 teaspoons baking soda

½ cup pitted and chopped cherries

2 cups shredded kale leaves

1 medium green apple, cored and chopped

½ cup shelled and crushed walnuts

In a blender, combine olive oil, baking soda, and cherries and blend until cherries are emulsified and all ingredients are thoroughly combined.

In a large bowl, combine the kale, apple, and walnuts, and drizzle the cherry oil over the top as desired.

Toss all ingredients until the salad is well dressed.

Place equal amounts of salad into two serving bowls. Serve immediately.

45: REMOVES RESIDUE FROM PRODUCE

Fruits and vegetables are usually shipped hundreds of miles from their points of origination to the grocery stores where we select the seemingly ripest and freshest varieties, but the average consumer is uneducated about the preservative processes that are involved in the growing and distribution processes of their produce. To help maintain and preserve the vibrant colors and textures that appeal to shoppers, farmers utilize countless pesticides and preservative sprays. These chemicals help produce keep their appealing appearance for days, weeks, and even months. With so many invisible, artificial substances added to produce, there are a number of hazardous health risks that can result from consuming unwashed fruits and vegetables.

In an attempt to consume a healthy diet rich in nutrient-dense foods, many consumers who are aware of produce residue try diligently to rinse and rid their produce purchases before preparing them for meals and snacks. Simply rinsing produce with soap and water can still leave traces of the chemicals on the surface of produce as well as within its permeable, porous layers. Luckily, baking soda has been heralded as one of the most effective produce cleansing agents that not only removes residue but also kills bacteria and microbes that can linger even after diligent washing and rinsing.

By combining 1 part baking soda and 2 parts water, the solution can be used as a soak or a spray to rinse produce thoroughly before it's eaten. With berries and soft produce being more porous, the soaking method should be utilized for up to 10 minutes before rinsing. Greens and cruciferous vegetables can be simply sprayed and rinsed without extended soaking periods.

46: MAKES A SKUNK DEODORIZER

Few odors compare to the overwhelming stench that a skunk can leave on skin and surfaces. The potent aroma can linger for days after a spray and serves as the skunk's defense mechanism against alarming situations and potential predators. People are often dumbfounded about how to rid themselves of the stench. While old wives' tales refer to tomato-based soaks and vinegar baths as successful ways to remove the smell of a skunk, few sufferers have actually found these methods to be worthwhile. Because the foul odor can seep into pores and infiltrate the skin's surface layers, a skunk stench can take days to alleviate.

However, baking soda eliminates the need for chemical-laden products and other questionable procedures because it combats the horrid odor of skunk stench naturally and effectively. By eliminating the caustic smell of the skunk's spray, baking soda provides the skin with pH-balancing detoxification that can help the body purge foreign substances and smells. With a soak that combines the natural relief of a pH-balancing product with a salt that extracts toxins and impurities, the skunk odor can not only be removed from the skin's surface, but the skin

and its underlying layers can receive therapeutic treatments that help heal and resist common agitations and irritations. A combination of 3 cups of baking soda and 4 cups of Epsom salt in a warm bath provides a soothing soak that cleanses and detoxifies, helping skunk-spray victims remedy their unpleasant odor.

In addition to the soak, an ingested tonic of 1 teaspoon of baking soda and ½ teaspoon of activated charcoal powder in an 8-ounce glass of water consumed three times daily can help purge the body of excessive toxins such as those deposited on the skin from a skunk spray. Repeating these implementations may not provide immediate relief but will shorten the duration of the residual skunk smell naturally and effectively.

47: BECOMES A DRY BATH FOR PETS

When your furry friends need a bath, but there's no access to water or your regular bathing supplies, what's an owner to do? With countless products on the market that cater to this precise predicament, it can be a dizzying process trying to determine which product is best for your pet. Many of these products promise to leave your pet feeling refreshed without drying or irritating their skin, but the chemicals and additives in these products can leave residues and produce drying effects on the animal's skin that lead to itchiness or irritation. The result of these side effects can be annoying and even dangerous for pets because constant scratching can lead to skin flare-ups while irritation can lead to catastrophic hair loss, skin conditions, and infection.

Luckily, baking soda provides pet owners with an all-natural alternative that has proven to be safe and effective for dogs and cats for decades. With an alkalizing benefit, baking soda can be utilized as a soothing application that not only restores pH balance to skin but also deodorizes the hair and skin without producing the drying effects of many other chemical-laden products. After ensuring that your pet's coat is completely dry (to prevent clumping and moisture residue), you can sprinkle baking soda on the surface of a dog's or cat's coat and simply smooth it into the hair and throughout the skin's surface. Once the baking soda has been evenly distributed throughout the coat, simply brush the hair to remove excess baking soda powder. Once the process is complete, there is no risk associated with your dog or cat scratching, fluffing, or licking the treated areas because of baking soda's safe, harmless, neutralizing effects. Some owners have even reported that their pets had better-smelling breath as a result of licking their baking soda–treated coats.

DOG-SWEAT SMELL

Whether your pooch suffers from stinkiness because he hasn't been bathed in a while or because your furry friend has been enjoying an afternoon of running around and playing catch, the smell of dog sweat can be a pungent odor. Much like dry shampoo often used by humans between showers, dry shampoo products for pets can have undesirable effects or contain harsh chemicals. With a quick application of baking soda on your pet's coat, the sweat smell can be minimized or eliminated safely and easily in just a matter of minutes.

48: MAKES A NATURAL PET RINSE

As with most pet products, the variety of wet pet-bath options can be astounding. The staggering number of treatments that cater to dry skin, irritated skin, itchiness, redness, hair loss, bites, fleas and ticks, and countless other conditions result in a plethora of products that promise to provide relief with "all-natural" or "organic" ingredients. But these same products can also contain harsh additives, chemicals, and questionable preservatives. Like people, pets have unique skin types that vary from dog to dog and cat to cat, so choosing the right product for your pet requires previous knowledge of their tolerance regarding synthetic ingredients. Another concern when choosing your wet bath products is that shampoos and conditioners that promise to moisturize can leave a film and residue on your pet's coat that they can ingest over time as they lick and scratch. This gradual consumption directly impacts the pH balance of your pet's mouth and body, making them susceptible to bad breath, illness, and a myriad of chronic conditions that sometimes include food aversion when their ability to taste is affected. Luckily, baking soda can be used as a wet-bath alternative to the chemical-laden soaks and rinses offered in stores.

With a pH-balancing effect, alkalizing baking soda can be combined with a simple solution of water and aloe for maximum benefit to both pet and owner. To eliminate the risk of harsh chemicals and additives on the skin's surface, a pet owner can combine ¼ cup of water, ½ cup of baking soda, and 2 cups of aloe vera to create a thick cleanser that can be applied without concern for gloves (or exposed wounds, since the cleanser poses no infection risk). The application should be smoothed onto the wet surface of the animal's coat, massaged throughout the fur, and rinsed thoroughly.

49: TREATS PET ACCIDENTS

Every pet owner knows that accidents happen. Whether it's a puppy learning curve, a delayed walk, a moment of fear, a display of territorial behavior, or a chronic condition affecting urination, pet accidents can occur at any time. Knowing this, pet supply companies market thousands of items that promise to rid your carpets and upholstery of stains and smells. These products are questionable for a number of reasons. Not only can chemical cleaners leave films and residues on carpets and upholstery that have the potential to adversely affect the skin and airways of both humans and pets, but stains can also be exacerbated by chemical interactions with certain fibers and colors, resulting in discoloration or "burns." Odors that pets leave behind might be successfully masked by products that only treat the smell of urine, but they still leave pets with a marked territory that *they* can smell, designating the area as one where they can return to relieve themselves regularly.

With a simple, safe, inexpensive one-to-one ratio of water and baking soda, this solution can be applied to any affected fabric or carpet by rubbing or brushing it into the fibers, allowing it to set for a period of 10–20 minutes, and then vacuuming it away. With an alkalizing effect that not only combats odors but also neutralizes the ammonia in urine, these treated areas will no longer have the "mark" of an area for urination. As an added benefit, the baking soda solution poses no risk of dying or bleaching treated areas, so carpets and upholsteries remain safe from stains and discoloration. As a safe alternative to chemical-laden products, baking soda provides pet owners with an inexpensive and effective accident treatment application that can be used anytime, anywhere.

50: CLEANSES PETS' TEETH AND GUMS

With oral hygiene playing such an essential role in maintaining the health of the entire human body, it only stands to reason that the same goes for pets. When pet breath makes snuggling with your favorite furry friend nearly unbearable, it can be tempting to seek relief in any one of the countless oral hygiene rinses that the major pet product manufacturers sell. However, many of these rinses, solutions, toothpastes, and even water additives that promise to help alleviate foul-smelling breath and restore health to your pet's mouth contain questionable ingredients that can aggravate the teeth, gums, and tongue while possibly exacerbating the underlying issues that cause bad breath and plaque buildup to begin with.

Since baking soda is safe and chemical-free, it's the perfect alternative to commercial oral hygiene products for pets. Homemade baking soda applications can be administered to dogs and cats alike without fear of damaging their overall health. A simple combination of 1 teaspoon of baking soda and 1 teaspoon of water can be used as a paste that's safe enough to brush the teeth, scrape the tongue, and rinse bacteria from the gums. This application can be performed once per week or as little as once per month to help your pet maintain clean teeth and gums that are free of plaque and bacteria. In addition, 1 teaspoon of baking soda can be added to your pets' water dish in order to target the foul, odor-producing bacteria that can linger in the mouth and digestive tract between brushings. With a small addition of 1 teaspoon of this alkaline powder, any pet owner can help prevent underlying health issues that could plague a pet's body...all by balancing their internal pH. Safe, inexpensive, and effective, baking soda provides the perfect dental health solution for your pet.

51: DEODORIZES AND CLEANS LITTERBOXES

While litterboxes are a convenient and self-contained area that can be concealed in almost any room of the house, they can create a foul-smelling aroma that permeates even the cleanest of homes. Specialized litters promise to trap odors in their crystals or mask unpleasant smells in other unique ways, but these odor-eliminating features can compromise the health of felines. Chemicals, additives, preservatives, and toxic substances can lurk in the litterbox of your precious pets, exposing them to a hazardous environment every time they step into the litter. Dangerous reactions triggered by the ammonia in urine coming in contact with the other chemical components of some litters can occur, leaving a toxic residue on a cat's feet and fur that is later consumed when he licks himself clean. Once these hazards are in a cat's mouth, they move through its digestive system and are quickly dispersed throughout its body, resulting in internal disturbances that can lead to the destruction of the cat's cells, organs, and systems.

By using baking soda to regularly clean and deodorize the litterbox, a cat owner can enjoy an odor-free environment that also doesn't pose a threat to their favorite furry friends. Sprinkling baking soda in an all-natural litter creates a disinfected space that not only combats bacteria and microbes but also neutralizes the source of odors. Simple, easy, and inexpensive, 1 tablespoon of baking soda can be sprinkled over the top of every fresh change of litter. An additional tablespoon of baking soda can be combined with ¼ cup of water to create a disinfecting rinse that helps clean and deodorize a litterbox. Once the application is applied, simply rinse, dry, and fill with new litter.

52: TREATS NAIL BLEEDING IN PETS

When a pet's nails get to a certain length, it is absolutely imperative to trim them. With every step, a pet's lengthy nails can wreak havoc on the pads of its feet, the tendons, the muscles in the arms and legs, and even the blood flow throughout the limbs. By having to arch the paws to compensate for the lengthy nails' striking points when walking or running, cats and dogs with long nails can suffer pain due to the development of tendonitis, arthritis, and a number of other inflammatory conditions that impede optimal growth and healthy living. With chronic inflammation, catastrophic conditions not only cause disfigurement and pain but can also result in cellular changes that lead to cancers.

In an effort to protect your dog or cat, regular nail trimming must be an essential element of their grooming and care. Many pet owners opt to trim their pets' nails themselves with a manual trimming tool or at-home tool kit (such as a Dremel dog and cat nail grinder kit). When pets move or struggle to avoid getting their nails trimmed, the "quick" or vein that runs into each nail can be nicked easily. When the quick is cut, the pet may experience slight pain and bleeding. Because baking soda is able to combat infection naturally, provide pain relief, and assist in clotting, keeping a bowl of baking soda on hand can prove beneficial during nail-clipping sessions. Following each clip of a nail, the paw can be placed into the powder for immediate relief and germ-protection. To wrap a wounded nail, soak a piece of gauze in a mixture of 1 tablespoon of baking soda and 1 tablespoon of water. Fasten it to your pet's paw for 5–10 minutes.

53: RELIEVES PETS' BAD BREATH

Just like humans, pets require proper oral hygiene (including the maintenance of teeth, tongue, and gums) to ensure that plaque, gingivitis, and infections stay at bay. With a variety of oral products available to care for dogs' and cats' teeth, many pet owners eagerly seek out the latest devices, rinses, and pastes that promise to cleanse their precious pets' mouths. In addition to traditional mouth-cleansing products, pet product manufacturers have also developed toys and treats that promise to rid animals' mouths of harmful bacteria that can cause bad breath. Unfortunately, the effectiveness of each of these products is overshadowed by the constant concern of chemicals, additives, and other harmful elements that can adversely impact pets' health and well-being. While these foul-breath treatments, toys, and treat products can quickly remedy bad breath, a pet owner has to keep in mind that consuming these products can also wreak havoc on the digestive system of pets, resulting in vomiting, diarrhea, and even difficulty passing bowel movements (especially if bits of undigested toys and treats linger in the digestive system).

In order to keep dogs and cats safe while attempting new treatments to remedy bad breath, pet owners should always opt for a safe, chemical-free rinse, paste, or water additive. This is exactly what baking soda offers. Mixing 1 teaspoon of baking soda into every cup of water in a pet's water dish can help cleanse his digestive system, return his pH to normal for optimal healing and health, and resolve any underlying issues that could be contributing to his bad breath problem. Also, pet owners can combine a one-to-one ratio of baking soda and water to make a toothpaste that removes plaque and bacteria, prevents infection, and (of course) remedies bad breath!

PART 2

BEAUTY

When you are tired of wasting money on chemical-laden products for your face, skin, and hair, look no further than a simple box of baking soda. Whether your concern is calluses, heavy residue in your hair, or an itchy skin condition, you can use one of the following amazing baking soda applications as a remedy. If you feel like your skin is succumbing to seasonal changes, a quick baking soda salve can help! If you're noticing that your hair feels weighed down during a blowout, baking soda can help!

With the dirt-cheap application of baking soda and water, you can transform the appearance of almost every area of your body. Whether it's rejuvenating your skin, adding volume to your hair, or alleviating health conditions that can affect everything from your eyes to your teeth, there's an easy-to-make, do-it-yourself baking soda application that can take the place of questionable and pricey commercial beauty solutions. Filled with effective applications that are free of odors, chemicals, and additives, this section's amazing tips and tricks will show you how to maximize the benefits of baking soda so you look and feel great every day!

54: RELIEVES ECZEMA

Millions of patients suffer from serious skin conditions each year, and a seemingly simple rash or irritation that can appear insignificant to many patients has the potential to develop into a severe problem. A simple scratch, bump, or even insect bite can transform a minor irritation into a more severe condition over the course of a few short hours or days. With conditions like eczema that exacerbate and complicate the skin's reaction to environmental toxins and microbial infestations, a minor skin condition can quickly transform into an itchy, red, inflamed rash. Uncomfortable, unsightly, and extremely difficult to resolve, eczema is another chronic skin condition that pharmaceutical companies have profited from with myriad creams, ointments, and salves that can cost tens to hundreds of dollars with no guarantee of relief.

There are countless medications and medicated creams that promise to provide relief from isolated or chronic flare-ups, but eczema can be a frustrating issue that presents itself any time an irritant triggers a rash to appear. Between the redness, itchiness, and discomfort, eczema can wreak havoc on everyday life. With countless products that promise to provide relief, eczema sufferers tend to treat their skin irritations with various pills and potions from the drugstore or grocery store, often to no avail. The problem is that these over-the-counter treatments contain synthetic ingredients and additives that can cause more harm than good.

Eczema sufferers should look to baking soda as an all-natural alternative to the potentially harmful synthetic remedies. A simple homemade treatment that consists of 1 part baking soda and 2 parts water can be applied as a natural remedy to any affected area. You'll reap the benefits of this anti-inflammatory, antibacterial, and antimicrobial solution, finding relief from the symptoms of eczema and restoring the body's pH balance, which is imperative to overall health and eczema recovery.

55: SOOTHES SUNBURNS

Sunburns seem to be a commonly accepted consequence of too much sun exposure. While these seemingly "normal" skin afflictions strike an alarming percentage of the population, the health consequences that can result from these periods of excessive sun exposure include major skin issues, such as skin cancer, later in life. While many companies try to capitalize on fears of skin cancer by providing plentiful products that promise to safeguard the skin from the sun's harmful rays, few provide adequate safety and security from sun exposure. These products that claim to safeguard the skin from the sun's damaging UVA and UVB rays contain countless chemicals and synthetic ingredients that can exacerbate chronic skin conditions or even intensify sunburns.

When a sunburn does occur, the most effective healing treatment contains baking soda! With an anti-inflammatory effect that also helps regulate and balance the body's pH, baking soda can help relieve the pain of sunburns while protecting the skin's cells from cancerous mutations that can be life-altering and life-threatening.

Whenever a sunburn is sustained, a simple solution of 1 part baking soda and 1 part aloe vera can be applied to the skin's surface and wrapped with gauze for a period of 1 hour. After the hour is up, the applications should be washed off with tepid water. Additionally, a bath soak that consists of 1 cup of baking soda and 1 cup of aloe vera can be utilized for immediate all-over relief and protection against harmful cellular changes. Soak for about 15–20 minutes and then let yourself air dry so as not to wipe the baking soda off.

56: SOFTENS HANDS

Between harsh environments, constant hand washing, and chemical-laden cleansers, it's no wonder that people are suffering from dry, cracked hands. Anyone who regularly does manual work and feels the pain and discomfort of irritated fingers, palms, and hands knows that the drying of these essential areas of the body can interfere with even the simplest movements and tasks. Regardless of the reasons for why or how this condition occurs, dry hands need tender love and care in order to be repaired. Cosmetic manufacturers provide consumers with a dizzying number of products that promise to return hardened hands to their supple original state, but it can be difficult to differentiate between quality products that will help from those that may cause more chaffing, dryness, and hardening of the skin. Luckily, baking soda can be used in a simple solution that can be combined with water and stored for use anywhere, anytime.

Baking soda has a pH-balancing, alkalizing effect that not only helps the internal aspects of the body but also improves the external condition of the skin. Soothing coconut oil that moisturizes and relieves irritation can be combined with baking soda and aloe vera to create a moisturizing application that can alleviate dryness due to exposure to the elements or harsh chemicals. By simply combining the following ingredients, anyone can create a hand-softening moisturizer that improves health, fights bacteria, and balances pH naturally!

TO MAKE THIS SOOTHING LOTION, COMBINE:

1 tablespoon baking soda
¼ cup aloe vera
¼ cup coconut oil

Combine the ingredients in a small bowl and apply to hands daily. The solution can be stored in an airtight container for up to 2 weeks.

BEAUTY BENEFITS OF ALL-NATURAL INGREDIENTS

With the implementation of certain ingredients, such as coconut oil and aloe vera, sensitive skin that reacts poorly to chemical-laden products can safely enjoy the same beautification results promised by synthetic brands. Do-it-yourself, at-home concoctions that include coconut oil and aloe vera, essential nutrients, healthy fats, and healing elements can not only help improve your skin's health but also improve its appearance with every use.

57: RELIEVES RASHES

Itchiness, redness, and scaly peeling skin can strike at any time of year and under any circumstances. Rashes can develop quickly due to weather and climactic changes or as a result of exposure or medication conflictions. Whether rashes result from myriad skin irritations, including exposure to harsh weather, chemicals, some insects, or certain kinds of foliage, the body is subjected to countless questionable elements that can compromise the immune system and the body's cells, organs, and systems.

Since the skin is the most vulnerable and susceptible organ of the body, people should always take precautions to safeguard it. While precautionary measures such as moisturizers, protective clothing, and avoiding certain elements can be taken, the skin can still experience unexpected and unexplained rashes. One way people can proactively prevent major skin problems is to quickly utilize natural healing remedies as soon as a skin irritation arises. In an attempt to address inflammation, redness, and itchiness, many people seek relief from creams, soaps, and soaks that promise to alleviate these symptoms and then fall victim to exacerbated skin conditions made worse by these chemical-laden products. Rather than applying unnatural products that can contain questionable ingredients and additives, a simple paste made with baking soda and aloe vera can be applied to the affected area of the skin for soothing relief of inflammation and regeneration of damaged skin cells. Adding to baking soda's ability to regulate pH and protect skin's cellular integrity, aloe vera is able to provide soothing vitamins and minerals that not only help revive skin but also deliver essential vitamins and minerals that are required for skin health.

TO MAKE THE PASTE, FOLLOW THESE STEPS:

1 tablespoon baking soda
2 tablespoons aloe vera

In a small bowl, mix the ingredients well and apply to the skin every 30–60 minutes until the rash subsides.

58: MAKES A NATURAL DEODORANT

With the frightening number of chemicals and synthetic additives that fill the average deodorant, many consumers are choosing to use all-natural alternatives. But the health-conscious consumer may find that she has few options when it comes to selecting an all-natural deodorant that is free of dyes, fragrances, and unnecessary chemicals. Certain seemingly safe ingredients are included in the formulation of most deodorants, but countless consumers have experienced adverse effects that include blocked sweat glands, decreased immunity, and even chronic illnesses. The "need" for deodorant has increased over time, but many hold steadfast in the belief that the body's organs and systems rectify the natural processes that lead to body odor if the body is allowed to function without intervention. Regardless of personal beliefs, it's wise for every consumer to take a critical look at what's in their deodorant. Knowing that anything put on the skin seeps into the bloodstream, deodorant users should choose their products wisely.

Because baking soda has an alkalizing effect, its pH-balancing power can eliminate odors naturally without interfering with the body's natural processes that release perspiration. Without chemicals and additives, a simple at-home application that uses baking soda as the active ingredient is an ideal alternative to chemical-filled, store-bought deodorants.

TO MAKE THE APPLICATION, FOLLOW THESE STEPS:

¼ cup baking soda
¼ cup coconut oil

In a small bowl, mix the ingredients well.

Once combined, the mixture can be poured into an ice cube tray and placed in the refrigerator to harden. After it's solidified, these convenient cubes can be stored in a cool, dark place, and used any time as a safe, chemical-free deodorant.

SWEET-SMELLING ADDITIONS

As you create your own do-it-yourself deodorants, you can customize the experience of wearing your new creation by including amazing natural aromas. As you combine the ingredients for your deodorant, add 1–20 drops of your favorite essential oil. Lavender, lemon, and eucalyptus are just a few examples of sweet-smelling additions that can improve your deodorant simply and easily.

59: CREATES A SOOTHING SOAK FOR IRRITATED SKIN

Skin irritation is a major concern for a growing percentage of the population. Whether the skin is sensitive due to genetics or a chronic condition, special care should be taken to ensure that skin irritations are limited as much as possible. Safeguarding the skin from chronic irritations such as environmental toxins, chemical-infused products, and everyday issues that can exacerbate sensitive skin issues can help minimize skin irritations. If these precautionary measures fail to protect the skin, there are countless products available that promise to provide relief. The issue with many of these products is that their ingredients can be more harmful than helpful. They are filled with synthetic ingredients that can cause skin irritations to worsen and spread. In fact, many of the over-the-counter skin irritant solutions can wreak havoc on the skin, creating more serious issues than the original irritation.

Baking soda can be used in a soothing bath soak to alleviate the common symptoms of skin irritations by providing the skin with anti-inflammatory benefits that immediately calm the reaction. By boosting the skin's immune response, baking soda can help reduce redness, itchiness, and swelling without any of the adverse side effects often induced by chemical-laden products.

Consumption of baking soda in a simple combination of 1 teaspoon of baking soda in an 8-ounce glass of water can help alleviate pH-balance related issues that can contribute to the skin irritations. In addition, by simply filling your tub with warm water and pouring in 1½–2 cups of baking soda, you can find immediate relief from skin irritation issues. This baking soda soak not only helps relieve the immediate irritation and inflammation, but it can also help prevent the onset of skin irritations in the future.

60: EXFOLIATES SKIN

As a multibillion-dollar per year industry, skin care products promise to reverse the signs of aging in specific regions of the face and body. These antiaging products make near-impossible promises, and it's no wonder that harsh chemicals and questionable additives grace the ingredient lists on the back of the bottles and jars. With no regard for the underlying issues that contribute to drying, sagging, and aging skin, many products simply moisturize but fail to deliver on their stated claims. For every area of rough skin, a different commercial treatment may be necessary, but baking soda can help alleviate all of those conditions easily, safely, and naturally.

Baking soda inherently possesses an all-natural pH-balancing effect that can rid the body's skin of excess oil or remedy dryness. With each application, baking soda can be used to improve the body's natural optimal balance, and with that balance comes a significant shift in skin health.

A simple combination of baking soda and other natural ingredients you probably already have at home can create a do-it-yourself exfoliant that not only moisturizes and rejuvenates the skin but also provides amazing benefits that improve its quality and protect its health. With each application scrubbed into the skin, dead cells can be removed and new skin cells are ushered in. By utilizing this simple solution, you can see immediate and progressive results that improve skin quality. With every use, the combination of beneficial ingredients helps improve and maintain the skin while preventing agitating or inflammatory conditions in the future.

TO MAKE THIS EXFOLIATING SCRUB, COMBINE:

1/8 cup baking soda

1/4 cup coconut oil

1/4 cup aloe vera

1 cup brown sugar

In a medium bowl, mix all the ingredients well.

Massage the scrub into the skin to remove dead skin cells.

Use this solution three or more times per week. The solution can be stored in an airtight container for up to 7 days.

61: TREATS DIAPER RASH

Countless moms around the country seek help in providing their babies with relief from diaper rash. In an occurrence of diaper rash, a child experiences pain and discomfort that can be compared to those experienced by an adult dealing with diarrhea or hemorrhoids. With several soothing applications available with prescriptions and over-the-counter products, it can be confusing as to which to use, how to apply, and how to alleviate the underlying issue.

Diaper rash usually occurs when a baby goes too long between diaper changes or when sensitivities to certain foods trigger diarrhea that results in a rash. The acidity of urine in particular can harm a baby's delicate skin and cause a red bumpy rash that is uncomfortable and sometimes painful. Chronic cases of this skin condition can adversely affect the growth and development of a young child, sometimes delaying certain milestones for months at a time. To exacerbate the situation, diaper rash can be intensified with over-the-counter treatments intended to alleviate the condition. Chemicals and synthetic additives intended to soothe the problem can actually worsen it. In lieu of these commonly prescribed ointments, many parents are looking for all-natural alternatives that can provide relief without the risk of adverse side effects.

With a simple sprinkle of baking soda on an irritated area, the risk of bacterial infection, inflammation, and pain are all reduced significantly. Any caregiver can make a simple paste made of 1 part baking soda and 1 part aloe vera that can be rubbed onto the affected skin area and left on for hours without concern. With pH-balancing effects that help combat the common symptoms of diaper rash, baking soda can help maintain optimal health by preventing future rashes from occurring.

62: SOFTENS FEET

With irritations and infections wreaking havoc on the health of patients with chronic foot conditions, it's no wonder why the beauty industry has cornered the market with a plethora of products that promise to provide relief for dry, cracked, and irritated feet. While these products can be effective to a certain extent, few fulfill their promise to permanently eliminate the pain and cure the underlying conditions that cause the issues in the first place.

When you seek a soothing footbath, you need look no further than the trusty box of baking soda inside your refrigerator door. Offering antibacterial, anti-inflammatory, and pH-balancing benefits, baking soda added to a soothing footbath not only fights pain, reduces redness, and combats inflammation but also improves circulation and helps maintain the quality of the skin on the feet. With every soak, baking soda's natural healing qualities nourish the feet with a boost of skin-protecting nutrients that fend off infection, promote healing, and help heal the chronic cracking and pain that can result from neglecting the skin on the soles of the feet.

To make a baking soda footbath, simply add 1 cup of baking soda to a 4-quart warm water footbath, to remedy your inflammation, irritation, and open wounds naturally. This all-natural approach not only remedies the symptoms of foot pain but also treats and cures its underlying causes, offering individuals a simple and inexpensive approach to ridding the chronic condition from their lives for good.

HARMFUL TOOLS FOR FEET

While it can be tempting to add pedicure tools such as pumices and scrapers in your foot-soothing and repairing routine, many studies have suggested that the use of these tools can actually contribute to the over-development of skin, leading to callused buildups of skin that have to be removed more frequently, or even wounds and infection. With soaking and gentle skin-removing techniques such as scrubs, the undesirable cycle of foot skin problems can finally come to a natural end.

63: MAKES A SOOTHING FOOTBATH

Whether you're a marathon runner, waitress, or just a busy parent on your feet all day, your feet can quickly and easily fall victim to soreness and irritation. When soothing socks, massaging rubs, and "organic" soaks fail to provide the relief you need, baking soda can deliver what other products and procedures can't: relief on the inside and out. With an internal relief of pH-balancing assistance that supports healthy nerve function, added to a soothing all-natural foot soak that provides topical relief to the layers of skin on the feet, baking soda can be the easiest and safest sore-foot savior.

Plentiful products promise to restore moisture, revitalize skin cells, and help repair damage that can result from simply walking too much every day, but it can be difficult to figure out the best remedy that will relieve the pains and aches while also rejuvenating the sore skin, muscles, and tendons of the feet. While many soaks claim to provide soothing restoration to tired feet, synthetic additives can result in excessive dryness, tenderness, and irritation, forcing consumers to sacrifice long-term help and healing in favor of immediate relief. With so much to be wary of, it's understandable that choosing

a footbath product can be difficult. While the majority of products can seem beneficial for foot health, careful consideration is required to determine which product's ingredients can improve health rather than hinder it.

However, an easy alternative is a simple solution containing ½ cup of baking soda, ½ cup of aloe vera, and ½ cup of coconut oil that creates the most soothing footbath imaginable. Penetrating deep within the skin's layers, aloe vera acts as a carrier for the anti-inflammatory baking soda. These two ingredients combine with coconut oil to promote a moisturizing benefit that helps restore a natural level of moisture while repairing damage done to the skin's surface. With no need for abrasive tools or treatments, this baking soda–based footbath allows feet to feel replenished and refreshed with no adverse health effects.

64: CREATES A THERAPEUTIC BODY SCRUB

With body scrubs becoming more commonly sought after, major manufacturers are producing countless varieties that promise to deliver unique benefits, specialized smells, and exfoliated, refreshed, and rejuvenated skin. These costly bath-time applications can leave you feeling tricked and teased, though. With harsh chemicals and abrasive additives that can actually leave your skin feeling dry or filmy, many of the body scrubs available today are riddled with ingredients that cause more harm than good. By choosing a skin-soothing body scrub that not only softens but also appeals to the senses, consumers can reap massive benefits, including improved skin health and minimized acne, blemishes, and discoloration. While many products on the market guarantee to provide these same benefits, few follow through. And, with a growing concern about the chemicals and additives that can dry skin, trigger irritations, and exacerbate existing issues, popular products have proven to be deceptive and downright unhealthy. With an at-home concoction that consists of baking soda and other all-natural ingredients, anyone hoping to achieve more beautiful, supple skin can find their new favorite body scrub in their very own kitchen cupboard.

Combining pH-balancing baking soda and essential oils such as lavender, eucalyptus, or lemon, with coconut oil greatly amplifies the health benefits these ingredients provide the skin. Evening out skin tone, minimizing irritation and inflammation, and providing the skin with essential moisturizers that are easily absorbed, this duo makes for a deeply nourishing, all-natural treatment. The addition of brown sugar not only helps create a euphoric experience for the senses, but it also provides the skin with a gentle exfoliate that removes dead skin cells without harsh abrasives. By combining each ingredient in equal parts, you can create your very own all-natural body scrub in the comfort of your own home.

65: REMOVES YELLOWING AND STAINS FROM NAILS

Countless scenarios can lead to yellowing of the nails, and baking soda has become one of the most popular and effective treatments among consumers to alleviate this problem. Whether the yellowing is a result of smoking, cooking with turmeric, or dealing with a wide variety of chemicals or dyes, this discoloration of the nails can be unsightly. While gloves can and should be worn when contact with these substances is anticipated, yellow, discolored nails can sometimes be unavoidable. It is surprising how persistent the yellow coloring can be at resisting nail polish remover and other alcohol-based products intended for stain removal. Luckily, the simple application of a baking soda treatment can remove yellow stains from nails while also naturally improving their health and growth.

Combining ¼ cup of baking soda with ½ cup of water creates a simple paste that can be applied to the nails. Whether you prefer to soak the nails by submerging them in the mixture or you feel more comfortable painting the treatment onto the nails, this naturally abrasive (yet nontoxic) combination removes the yellow stain from nails without the use of chemicals, additives, or harsh and harmful ingredients. Proven to be effective, inexpensive, and simple, this easy paste can be applied as often as necessary to ensure that nails stay free of discoloration. As an added benefit, the combination of pH-balancing baking soda and purified water helps stimulate the growth of healthy cells within the skin and nails, resulting in stronger, longer, healthier nails that resist breaking. Natural, safe, and effective, this simple baking soda combination can be used by anyone in search of a better way to achieve dye-free nails that are healthier with every single treatment.

66: MAKES AN EASY PRE-MANICURE TREATMENT

The condition of a person's nails can speak loudly about their profession, devotion to care for themselves, and much more. With everyday activities that range from typing to gardening to washing dishes, it can be easy to have nails, nail beds, and cuticles fall victim to careless neglect. One of the easiest ways to maintain nail health, reduce the risk of infection and inflammation, and prepare for perfect-looking hands and feet is baking soda.

Every year, consumers pay billions of dollars on manicures. While this seemingly insignificant expense might seem frivolous to some, the ideal manicured look is worth the expense to many others. The manicure market is being cornered by shops that provide services at relatively low prices, and the demand for manicures refuses to budge even in poor economic environments.

While manicuring kits are readily available at local drug stores or specialty beauty stores, many people opt for the full-service salon experience— from which they leave with perfectly manicured fingernails that glisten and glow without chips or flaws. However, if salon services are unattainable, and the do-it-yourself manicure is your only option, it can be tempting to simply file, buff, and paint. But a quick and easy pre-manicure treatment that contains baking soda as its star ingredient can make a do-it-yourself manicure look just like the salon version…without an excessive commitment of time or money.

Simply combine ¼ cup of baking soda with ½ cup of coconut oil and apply the treatment to your nails and cuticles, brushing delicately with a soft paintbrush or toothbrush. Once the nails and cuticles are fully prepped, you can apply your base coat, nail color, and topcoat to achieve a long-lasting manicure that will look beautiful (and professionally done) for far longer than a manicure that hasn't been prepped thoroughly with baking soda.

67: SOFTENS CALLUSES

Regardless of your profession, unsightly calluses can develop on your hands and feet. The working mom who constantly washes dishes and delves into household chemicals has the same issues as the mechanic or industrial worker: irritants and abrasives cause skin cells to accumulate on the surfaces as a natural form of protection. The bad news is that this accumulation develops into the unsightly calluses.

Whether they form as a result of manual labor, overworking a specific area of the skin, or excessive rubbing, calluses can be uncomfortable and unsightly. Any one of an assortment of chronic skin conditions can also lead to this minor disfigurement of the hands and feet. Calluses can be an annoying disruption to the normal functioning of the extremities. Over time, calluses can become harder to remove and may become a permanent fixture that require surgical removal. In order to avoid the development of persistent calluses or the permanent hardening of specific areas affected by calluses, many over-the-counter products promise to provide the skin with softening benefits that help return it to normal. While these products may seem enticing, the truth is that the chemicals they contain can lead to serious skin conditions that result in overly sensitive, irritated, or inflamed areas.

Baking soda, on the other hand, can provide an all-natural, safe soak that can help rid the skin of hardened calluses simply and easily over time. By combining ¼ cup of baking soda with 2 cups of warm water, the afflicted areas of the hands or feet can be soaked for 15–30 minutes once to three times daily, softening the skin naturally. Following the soak, you should use a pumice stone to gently remove hardened, dead skin layers. Following this routine, your callus-ridden areas can be returned to healthy, supple, conditioned skin within a matter of days or weeks…without the agitation or irritation that can accompany chemical-laden, commercial alternatives.

68: BECOMES A SPOT-TREATMENT FOR ACNE

Acne is one of the most prevalent skin conditions that occurs in every population, regardless of sex, age, or race. There are countless contributing factors that lead to the development of acne, and it can sometimes be difficult to pinpoint the specific condition or situation that triggers every unsightly breakout. Acne can appear on skin in isolated areas throughout the face, neck, back, arms, and chest, making treatment a difficult process. Pharmaceutical companies have developed a plethora of harsh medications that promise to provide relief, competing with millions of manufactured over-the-counter rinses, washes, and creams that can be used in a number of acne-fighting routines. As with many processed treatment methods, though, these applications often contain harsh chemicals and additives that not only fail to rid the skin of acne but also exacerbate the problem, resulting in further irritation and inflammation. Luckily there are all-natural alternatives that can be crafted at home to treat the surface of the skin while also returning the body's systems to optimal health.

Ingesting a daily dose of 1 tablespoon of baking soda dissolved in an 8-ounce glass of water can provide your body with pH-balancing benefits that can help rid the body's systems naturally of toxins, correct hormonal imbalances, and metabolize nutrients efficiently. In addition to ingesting dissolved baking soda, a rinse of 1 part baking soda and 2 parts water can be used in the shower or bath twice daily to help return the skin to a balanced pH level. For spot treatments of acne, a one-to-one ratio of baking soda and water can be applied as a paste to the afflicted areas three times a day and left to remain on the skin for 30 minutes at a time before rinsing. With these three applications that contain potent, pH-balancing baking soda, any acne sufferer can find relief from unsightly blemishes while preventing further outbreaks in the future.

69: MAKES A NATURAL FACE CLEANSER

A simple stroll down the skin care aisle of a drug store or your favorite corner market will probably reveal an overwhelming selection of facial cleansers. Finding the perfect all-natural facial cleanser that doesn't contain excessive chemicals or additional agents can be difficult. However, anyone seeking to safely and naturally cleanse their face can find peace of mind and relief in a matter of minutes with a simple at-home, do-it-yourself combination of all-natural ingredients.

This face cleansing creation utilizes baking soda's neutralizing pH properties to help restore a homeostatic balance that improves skin health while also minimizing irritation, inflammation, and redness, as well as eliminating excessive dryness or oiliness.

Three simple, all-natural ingredients will help extract dirt from pores, mildly exfoliate dead skin cells, and moisturize the multiple layers of the skin—all while safely removing dirt and grime. This solution provides the skin with ample benefits that replenish the skin's health without posing any risk to those with sensitive skin or serious skin issues. This baking soda–based face cleanser is an amazing, all-natural alternative for people seeking a simple cleansing solution that can be made in the comfort of their own home.

TO MAKE THIS CLEANSER, FOLLOW THESE STEPS:

¼ cup baking soda

1 tablespoon brown sugar

½ cup aloe vera gel

Combine the ingredients in a medium bowl and apply to the face with the fingertips or a soft cloth. Massage the mixture into the skin for 1–2 minutes before rinsing with warm water.

RECOMMENDATIONS FOR USE:

Recommended for use twice daily. It is safe enough for use as often as necessary. Any remaining solution should be stored in an airtight container for up to 1 week.

70: CREATES A FACE MASK FOR OILY SKIN

With skin health being at the forefront of your personal presentation, it's no wonder that the skin care industry makes up a significant portion of the billions of dollars spent by consumers annually. Both women and men are increasingly interested in the latest and greatest products that promise to deliver the clearest skin. Not surprisingly, baking soda can be used to provide this too.

The skin's surface is made up of multiple layers that each contain glands. Sebaceous glands work hard to ensure that sweat is released without issue, that pores aren't riddled with dirt and grime, and that the perfect balance of oils and dryness ensures the skin's optimal health. While it's true that natural oils are needed to keep the skin's surface from over-drying and becoming jeopardized by the environment, changes in climate, and toxins, some people have skin that's too oily and can prove to be problematic. With excessive oil on the face, pores are unable to "breathe" and can become overwhelmed with dirt particles, leading to blackheads. This excess oil can also lead to the development of inflammation,

irritation, and acne. Using simple cleansers (as detailed in the previous entry) and the following baking soda–based face mask, anyone can create their own all-natural, oil-removing face products right in their own home. This mask will help remove toxins, dirt, grime, buildup, and irritants on a regular basis and can be used nightly.

TO MAKE THE FACE MASK, FOLLOW THESE INSTRUCTIONS:

¼ cup baking soda
1 tablespoon activated charcoal powder
¼ cup aloe vera gel
1 tablespoon lemon juice

In a small dish, combine all ingredients and mix thoroughly.

Using your fingertips, apply the mask to the skin with gentle circular motions until the entire surface of the face is coated.

Allow the mask to set for 10–15 minutes before rinsing with warm water.

RECOMMENDATIONS FOR USE:

Use as often as every night until excessive oil production is diminished.

71: WORKS AS A NATURAL HAND SOAP

Among the countless products that promise to help retain beauty while preserving health are a variety of hand soap products that claim to keep your skin healthy throughout dishwashing, weather changes, and excessive hand washing. While manufacturers promote their own ingredients as being "all-natural," "organic," or without artificial additives, these hand soaps are rarely as natural as they seem. In order to combat bacteria and microbes, many hand soaps add harsh additives and synthetic antimicrobial combatants that can dry out skin. Moisturizers are added to counterbalance the drying effect, but many hand soaps can leave your hands feeling slimy or covered with an obvious oily film as a result. For consumers who seek a truly all-natural alternative to commercial hand soaps, the following baking soda–based hand soap combines pH-balancing baking soda, microbial-combatting citrus juice, and moisturizing aloe vera to ensure that hands are cleansed of germs and toxins, protected against skin conditions such as irritation and inflammation and nourished with natural moisturizers that help retain skin's suppleness.

With the following recipe you can quickly and easily make a soap that will contribute to the health of your hands while also safeguarding against irritation, inflammation, illness, disease contraction, the manifestation of chronic conditions, and premature aging. You can use this soap as often as necessary throughout the day or night, and it can be stored in an airtight container to be taken to work, school, or on a trip to ensure that your hands receive the protection they need and the care and attention they deserve. This sensitive-skin solution helps maintain optimal health of the entire body while fighting common conditions that can compromise the skin health of the hands.

TO MAKE THE HAND SOAP, FOLLOW THESE STEPS:

2 tablespoons baking soda
2 tablespoons lemon juice
¼ cup aloe vera gel

In a small bowl, mix all the ingredients well.

Store in an airtight container and use as often as needed.

72: RELIEVES TOENAIL FUNGUS

Fungal infections are far more prominent than many people believe. Moist, dark environments provide fungi with ample growth opportunities, so it's no wonder that sweaty feet can be the perfect breeding ground for fungus. With regular washing, allowance for ample air exposure, and decontamination with natural treatments, many fungal infections can be prevented naturally, but if you find yourself dealing with the unexpected onset of a fungal infection in the toenails, you should take immediate action.

With the itchiness, inflammation, irritation, discoloration, and foul-smelling odors that can all result from fungal infections of the toenails, it's not surprising that pharmaceutical companies and over-the-counter product manufacturers offer many solutions for the issue. While these medications and treatments seem promising when it comes to providing relief, the chemicals and additives that they contain can lead to an exacerbation of the toenail fungus that can permanently disfigure the feet and toes if left untreated.

Because baking soda has the ability to balance pH levels, it can shift the environment that previously allowed toenail fungus to thrive to one that combats its growth and rids the skin and nails of the spores altogether. With a simple footbath that combines 1 part baking soda and 2 parts warm water, any foot fungus sufferer can stop the growth of fungus while also providing the feet with the pH balance required to safeguard against future fungal infections. This soothing foot soak can also be utilized as a preventative measure that also provides curative properties…all while therapeutically treating the senses as well.

73: REMEDIES BLACKHEADS NATURALLY

Everyday activities can contribute to the buildup of toxins, dirt, and grime that can get trapped in the skin's pores. Not only can these blocked pores inhibit the natural excretion of toxins and the body's normal sweat, but the trapped buildup can also lead to the development of blackheads. When the skin has substances trapped within its surface without any way of purging the pores, pimple-like developments arise on the skin's surface and appear black. While acne and whiteheads can be irritating, unsightly, and uncomfortable, blackheads can be more difficult to deal with because they result from deeply imbedded buildup in the skin's subsurface pores. By trying to rid the skin of these blackheads by poking, prodding, and popping, any blackhead sufferer can find themselves dealing with major skin irritations, inflammation, or permanent scarring. With an all-natural recipe that utilizes the cleansing power of baking soda, anyone who wants to get rid of blackheads can do so simply, easily, and naturally.

Baking soda has the amazing ability to balance the pH of the skin while ridding the body of toxins and bacteria that can contribute to the buildup that causes blackheads. With a simple rinse of a baking soda–based solution that consists of 1 part baking soda and 2 parts water, the skin can be refreshed and replenished, freeing the pores of residue…all while improving the skin's ability to naturally combat the buildup. With the wash applied, a gentle scrub with the fingertips and a thorough rinse with warm water can help resolve blackheads naturally. In addition, you can make the following topical application to extract toxins, impurities, and foreign elements that can become trapped in the skin.

TO MAKE A BLACKHEAD-COMBATTING APPLICATION, SIMPLY TAKE:

1 teaspoon baking soda
1 teaspoon activated charcoal powder
1 tablespoon water

In a small bowl, mix the ingredients until they form a paste.

Apply to the blackhead-affected area and massage the paste gently into the skin with your fingertips. Rinse thoroughly with warm water.

74: BRIGHTENS SKIN

Countless consumers seek out products that promise to provide their face and skin with a sun-kissed glow. Whether they be moisturizers, rinses, masks, or other applications, these products often contain chemicals, additives, or ingredients that can strip the natural layers of the skin in order to give the impression of a lustrous "glow." While the immediate result may be glowing skin, the hidden dangers lie in the consequences of removing layers of the skin with questionable chemicals and synthetic substances. The visual benefit of glowing skin is often accompanied by unpleasant residual effects that include irritation, inflammation, redness, and acne. While you may achieve a temporary glow with the simple application of an over-the-counter treatment, the long-term effects of these applications can be detrimental to the health of your skin for years, if not a lifetime.

In order to avoid damaging, artificial ingredients, many consumers have sought out all-natural alternatives to brighten, rejuvenate, and cleanse their skin, unclog their pores, and bring the body's pH into balance. One of the most effective natural ingredients that provides all these benefits is baking soda. Without risking the health of the skin or contributing to the development of serious skin issues, baking soda can be used in combination with other all-natural ingredients to create a scrub that gives you a healthy glow while also improving and maintaining your skin's well-being.

TO MAKE THIS SIMPLE SCRUB, FOLLOW THESE STEPS:

1 tablespoon baking soda
2 tablespoons lemon juice
¼ cup water
¼ cup aloe vera gel

In a medium bowl, mix the ingredients well.

Massage into the skin and rinse off with warm water to reveal glowing skin.

RECOMMENDATIONS FOR USE:

This scrub can be used as often as three times a day. The solution can be stored in an airtight container for up to 7 days.

75: REMOVES SPRAY TAN/FAKE TAN

With awareness increasing about the sun's damaging effect to the skin's surface and delicate cells within the skin's multiple layers, a growing percentage of the population is seeking alternatives to the glorious glow of a sun-kissed tan. Informed individuals are making an effort to minimize their risk of developing serious skin conditions such as sunburns, irritations, rashes, inflammation, redness, or even cancerous growths. With these legitimate concerns making sun exposure a questionable endeavor, the many consumers who revel in the "healthy" glow of a suntan have turned to products and procedures that promise to provide a sun-kissed look without the dangers of actual sun exposure.

These creams, sprays, and salon treatments can provide consumers with their desired skin tone, but there are a number of problems associated with their use that can leave patrons with feelings of regret. Between artificial orange tones, streaks, and excessive discoloration throughout the body, a proportionate percentage of unhappy customers seek out an option that can remove the fake/false coloring. While normal showering, scrubbing, and soaking with traditional soaps and washes can't remove these dyes, there is an all-natural remedy that can be used to rid the skin of fake tanning products.

To naturally and safely remove your fake tan, fill a bathtub with warm water, 2 cups of baking soda, and 2 cups of apple cider vinegar and mix the ingredients thoroughly. Soak in the tub for 15–30 minutes, and then use a wash cloth or mildly abrasive towel to scrub the fake tanning solution from your skin. Following the soak and scrub, a simple rinse with warm water will help rid the skin of any lingering tanning solutions safely and naturally.

76: MAKES A NATURAL TOOTHPASTE

There is no question that the condition of the mouth can transform the health of the entire body. With proper care, the hygiene of the mouth translates into proper digestion, improved immunity, and optimal systematic functioning throughout the body. By contrast, a mouth that is poorly cared for gives a plethora of bacteria, viruses, fungal spores, and microbes the opportunity to riddle the body with multiple complications. With this information in mind, toothpaste manufacturers have developed countless products that promise to provide protection against gingivitis, irritations around the teeth and gums, and serious conditions that compromise the health of the teeth, tongue, cheeks, and throat.

While many of these toothpastes claim to rid the mouth of harmful bacteria and microbes while cleansing the teeth of harmful plaque and food residue, most of these products contain questionable ingredients that can exacerbate existing health issues in the mouth, increase tooth sensitivity, degrade the enamel on the surface of teeth, and compromise the healthy pH balance of the mouth.

Completely free of adverse side effects, 1 tablespoon of baking soda can be used in combination with ½ tablespoon of water and ½ tablespoon of coconut oil to create a paste that not only combats germs, microbes, and harmful bacteria but also extracts existing harmful organic elements with every brushing.

77: WHITENS TEETH

Nothing conveys beauty and a sense of attractiveness like a pearly white smile. Unfortunately, the constant barrage of staining drinks (like coffee and colas), poor habits (like smoking), and even medicinal side effects all contribute to the yellowing, browning, and greying of teeth, leaving many people seeking treatments that promise to deliver a sparkling white smile. While the pastes, strips, rinses, and light treatments that are available over the counter or in dental offices across the globe make teeth whitening seem like an easy, inexpensive, and common procedure, the truth is that many of these procedures come with serious long-lasting consequences. The chemicals and additives that wreak havoc on the base of the teeth and gums can lead to permanent conditions such as severe hot and cold sensitivity, recessed gum lines, and exposure of the nerves within teeth. These conditions can result in mouth pains and even susceptibility to cavities and unnecessary root canals.

With so much information available about the possible side effects associated with periodic or consistent use of chemical-laden teeth whiteners, many consumers are seeking out effective treatments that can provide desirable effects without undesirable side effects. Baking soda provides just that. You can make a simple at-home concoction of 1 tablespoon of baking soda and 1 tablespoon of water mixed into a paste. Apply the paste to your teeth and allow it to set for 10–15 minutes before brushing thoroughly. You can use this treatment up to twice a day if you desire. With added benefits that safeguard the mouth and the body's systems from harmful chemicals, this simple baking soda solution can be utilized as often as necessary, effectively producing desiring results without any health concerns whatsoever...for a mere cost of pennies per treatment!

78: ACTS AS A NATURAL MOUTHWASH

Mouthwashes litter the aisles of grocery stores, corner stores, and specialty stores, leaving customers and clients questioning which is the most beneficial. These plentiful products that promise to alleviate, rid, or prevent common dental hygiene issues with a simple swish can contain ingredients that not only irritate the teeth and gums but also rid the mouth and digestive system of beneficial bacteria. By counteracting the body's natural pH balance, bacterial balance, and homeostatic regularity, the common mouthwashes purchased by consumers can lead to more detriment than benefit.

Baking soda can be used as an all-natural alternative solution that not only rids the mouth of harmful bacteria and microbes but also promotes the proper pH balance required by the mouth and body. It also acts as a mild abrasive solution that is able to seep into the crevices between teeth and gums to ensure that cleansing those hard-to-reach areas is achieved with every use.

In addition to the plentiful, health-optimizing benefits of baking soda's pH-balancing capabilities, the inclusion of coconut oil to this daily swish has shown to provide significant improvements in gum health, retainment of tooth enamel, and the elimination of harmful bacteria while still retaining the mouth's beneficial bacteria. This mouth rinse will rid your mouth of plaque and harmful microbes and also improve your gum health and whiten your teeth in just a matter of 2 short weeks.

TO MAKE THIS MOUTH RINSE, FOLLOW THESE STEPS:

1 tablespoon baking soda
2 tablespoons coconut oil

Dissolve the baking soda into the coconut oil.

Swish the mouthwash around your mouth for 10–15 minutes and then spit it out.

RECOMMENDATIONS FOR USE:

Use this mouthwash twice a day for optimal results. The solution can be stored in an airtight container for up to 7 days.

79: MAKES A KID-SAFE CAVITY-FIGHTING MOUTH RINSE

Caring for children's teeth has always been a debate; whether the fight be between parents and their children at bedtime, dentists and the medical community about fluoride, or the questionable effects of certain medications on long-term teeth and gum health, there has always been an adversarial questioning relating to children's oral hygiene. To make matters even more confusing, a growing number of products appear on the market that promise parents to provide their children with "healthy" oral hygiene care.

With a growing concern about the ingredients in children's products, it only makes sense that mouthwashes, rinses, and swishes should come under careful scrutiny. Parents are often faced with choosing a fluoride-containing or fluoride-free mouth rinse while also trying to take into consideration taste and effective oral hygiene–promoting ingredients. All these choices can make the selection of kid-safe mouth rinses dizzying.

Widely accepted information shows that childhood dental hygiene plays a major role in overall health and development throughout life, so it's no wonder that the selection of oral hygiene products for children cause major concern for parents.

While the manufacturers of child-focused oral hygiene products have the market flooded with products that appeal with cartoon characters, "all-natural" labels, and claims of being free of harmful ingredients, the majority of these products contain questionable ingredients or have a taste that's undesirable to children.

By creating your own baking soda–based rinse, any parent can have their child utilize the cleansing powers of one of the most effective all-natural ingredients. With no concern for the adverse effects that can result from the questionable ingredients contained in store-bought mouthwashes, 1 tablespoon of baking soda can be dissolved in ¼ cup of lukewarm water to create a safe mouth rinse that not only naturally combats bacteria and fights plaque buildup but also promotes proper pH and is still palatable for the little ones in your life.

80: ELIMINATES BAD BREATH

The majority of consumers consider bad breath to be a condition that can be easily treated with a regular routine of brushing and mouthwash rinses. What many people fail to realize is that bad breath is rarely due to any condition of the mouth but is usually a direct reflection of the condition of the digestive system and related physical processes. When the body exhibits foul odors, whether through flatulence or foul-smelling breath, the odor is an indication of disrupted or malfunctioning digestive processes.

With plentiful products available that promise to provide the body with proactive enzymes, probiotics, and so on that can return your body to optimal health, there are few that actually deliver the health-optimizing benefits they claim. By choosing an all-natural alternative ingredient that can be utilized in a number of treatment methods, anyone suffering from bad breath can alleviate the condition naturally.

Baking soda can be consumed on a regular basis in a solution of 1 tablespoon of baking soda dissolved in 1 cup of water every morning. Not only does this solution help return the body to a balanced pH level that promotes proper digestion and hormonal functions for proper metabolism, but it also provides the body with a cleansing, alkalizing benefit that makes the body better able to process toxins and odor-producing components. In addition to the ingestion of baking soda, a mouth rinse that consists of 1 tablespoon of baking soda and 2 tablespoons of coconut oil can be used as often as desired throughout the day to rid the mouth of odor-producing bacteria and microbes. With this multifaceted approach to curing the underlying cause of bad breath, anyone suffering from the condition can utilize baking soda to rid themselves of the problem permanently.

81: REMOVES PLAQUE

Plaque buildup can happen with chronic unhygienic practices or a simple neglect of proper oral hygiene over time. Regardless of the cause, plaque buildup can be unsightly, unhealthy, and a threat to overall health. While the buildup of plaque can be an unobservable issue over time, the drastic consequences it can have on oral health, hygiene, and even chronic illness and disease is well documented and of serious concern. Science has shown that oral hygiene has a direct effect on overall health and well-being; luckily, baking soda can help!

While the majority of people are aware of the dangers that plaque can create, few can confidently say that they know what plaque is, how it deposits on the teeth, or what the consequences of excessive plaque deposits can be. Considering all the well-marketed products that promise to remove plaque, prevent plaque deposits, and return the mouth to optimal health, a staggering percentage of the population visits the dentist for a regular visit only to be told that their plaque buildup is still at a harmful concentration. These deposits can not only deteriorate and compromise the health of teeth but can contribute to mild conditions like bad breath and more serious conditions like gingivitis. Regardless of the severity of plaque buildup, anyone hoping to preserve their dental health, and their overall health, should incorporate a baking soda–based treatment in their everyday routine.

With a mildly abrasive texture, 1 teaspoon of baking soda can be combined with 1 teaspoon of coconut oil to create an all-natural toothpaste that can be used like the over-the-counter alternatives; helping to remove plaque, rid the mouth of bacteria and microbes, and restore a proper pH balance. This combination of ingredients helps maintain the optimal health of the teeth gums, tongue, and mouth without concern for chemicals, additives, or harsh ingredients that can all contribute to serious dental issues. Baking soda's natural abilities can return the mouth's environment to one that is not only able to prevent plaque buildup, but also promote health for the prevention of serious dental hygiene issues. Over-the-counter plaque-prevention products can't even compare to the effectiveness of baking soda.

82: SOOTHES RAZOR BURN

With every swipe of a razor, the possibility of developing "razor burn" is ever-present. The beauty industry preys on men and women who fear the unsightly and uncomfortable conditions that result from worn razors. Whether due to sensitive skin, persistent irritation, or a chronic skin condition that leaves the skin especially vulnerable, razor burn can strike anyone. While precautionary measures such as using fresh razors, using shaving cream while shaving, and shaving in specific directions on different parts of the body can all help reduce the incidence of razor burn, the condition can still occur. In an attempt to minimize razor burn, many commercial products promise that their formulas can be used before, during, or after shaving to prevent razor burns from occurring. Sadly, these products rarely help. Adding to the already uncomfortable skin irritation, the chemicals and additives in many of the creams, soaks, and lotions can further irritate inflamed areas. By blocking the hair follicles that become irritated during shaving, many products' residues can contribute to ingrown hairs that can be unsightly, uncomfortable, and even hazardous to your overall health.

Luckily, baking soda can be used in two separate methods for the prevention and treatment of razor burn. With a simple concoction created by combining 1 part baking soda and 1 part coconut oil, a soothing lather can be applied to the skin prior to shaving. Helping to reduce skin irritation and soothe areas of possible inflammation, a similar combination consisting of 1 part baking soda and 1 part aloe vera can be applied to skin post-shave. With the natural calming effects that are provided by the pH-balancing, alkalizing baking soda, these simple combinations of all-natural ingredients not only help maintain the suppleness of the skin, but also provide relief from the pain, itchiness, and redness that can occur from razor burn.

83: DETOXIFIES PORES

While the skin seems like a protective sheath that protects the body from harmful toxins and environmental filth, the skin's permeable layers are riddled with pockets of permeable funnels that not only allow the skin to breathe and expel waste, but can also become clogged with everyday substances that are in the air, are introduced through touch, and are deposited through contact of any kind. With this constant barrage of dirt, grime, and harsh elements, the detrimental exposure that the skin endures daily can be astounding. Anyone who fails to provide their skin with a detoxifying process every day only furthers the degradation of their skin's cells, thickening of the skin's layers, and toxic buildup that fills the skin's pores with unhealthy grit. Because the skin is one of the most sensitive organs, the entire surface of the body is susceptible to unimaginable toxicity that can transform a young, healthy body to one that is riddled with wrinkles, large pores, discoloration, and even serious health-complicating conditions such as cancer. With a natural approach to cleansing the skin that revolves around the benefits of baking soda, anyone can detoxify their skin safely, easily, and naturally.

With no need for abrasive products that contain harsh chemicals, a beauty routine that focuses on natural ingredients can not only help reduce the incidence of chronic skin conditions, but do so without the possibility of exacerbating inflammation, irritation, redness, acne, etc. With the implementation of baking soda's alkalizing benefits, anyone can not only improve the condition of their skin, but also reverse previous damage and prevent future damage.

Helping to detoxify the pores, purge toxins from the skin's surface, and protect the skin's cells against toxicity, a combination of 1 tablespoon of baking soda, ¼ cup of aloe vera, and ½ teaspoon of activated charcoal can be used as a daily treatment that is applied to the face, gently massaged into the skin's surface, and rinsed with lukewarm water.

84: MAKES A MOISTURIZING FACIAL SCRUB

As with most beauty products on the market, facial scrubs and cleansers are available for almost any specific need or concern imaginable. Whether your skin be blemished or sensitive, inflamed or riddled with acne, there are a plethora of skin care products that seem to have been designed just for you. While these seemingly helpful products may be enticing, the appeal of their marketing ploys can fall flat when it comes to your specific skin care needs. Oily, dry, irritated skin requires a balance with pH, not a "mask" that simply alleviates a skin issue for a few hours. Without the need of these over-the-counter scrubs that can irritate skin, cause inflammation, and exacerbate skin conditions, you can create your very own moisturizing facial scrub at home with a few simple ingredients that are probably in your cupboards and refrigerator right now.

Baking soda–based facial scrubs allow for the skin to be rejuvenated and refreshed by balancing the pH levels and alkalizing any acidity that lurks beneath the skin's surface. With the addition of coconut oil and aloe vera for deep penetrating moisture for the skin's many layers, the skin is not only replenished but also safeguarded against harmful toxins and carcinogens. Adding brown sugar allows for the scrub to be mildly abrasive without damaging the skin's surface or adding any chemical-laden additives that can irritate or inflame the skin.

TO MAKE THIS FACIAL SCRUB, FOLLOW THESE STEPS:

1 tablespoon baking soda
⅛ cup coconut oil
⅛ cup aloe vera gel
2 tablespoons brown sugar

Combine the ingredients in a small bowl and mix together well.

Apply the mixture to the face and massage it in gently to ensure all areas are treated.

Rinse with warm water and follow your normal beauty routine as usual.

RECOMMENDATIONS FOR USE:

This application can be used twice daily, or as needed.

85: SOOTHES TATTOO APPLICATIONS

The tattoo industry is booming with new and exciting approaches to the application of these permanent markings, and countless consumers seek out the artistic gifts of talented artists each and every day. While many of these artists are masters of their work, there is always the possibility that errors, accidents, or injuries can occur in the tattooing process. Even if these conditions aren't apparent at the time of the tattoo's application, the symptoms of infection or injury can slowly appear over the course of the days following the procedure. Redness, scabbing, inflammation, heat, swelling, and pain all signifying the body's adverse reaction to the tattoo, whether due to the repetitive insertion of the needle or the dye used in the tattoo's design, it is imperative to remain aware of the symptoms that may indicate a health-compromising issue in order to apply or seek out necessary treatment options as soon as possible.

While few people fail to recognize the serious consequences of skin irritations that result from permanent tattoos, the health complications are all too real. From irritations to infections to serious blood complications, the irritations and inflammation resulting from a tattoo can be catastrophic. Fortunately, baking soda can help!

Luckily, one of the most effective treatments that can be used to ensure infection, irritation, and inflammation do not occur at the site of a new tattoo is a baking soda application.

TO MAKE THIS SOOTHING PASTE, USE:

1 part baking soda
1 part aloe vera

Mix the ingredients together to form a paste.

Apply to the area of the new tattoo and allow to set for 10–15 minutes before rinsing with warm water.

RECOMMENDATIONS FOR USE:

This application can be used as often as necessary throughout the days following the tattoo application until the healing has completed.

86: REDUCES WRINKLES

Wrinkles are an inevitable appearance on the skin as we age. With genetics, health habits, and exposure to certain elements all contributing to the development and severity of wrinkles, it can be difficult to control their onset and extensiveness. Like many aspects of aesthetics, wrinkles are one of the most prominently addressed issues in the beauty industry. There are hundreds of creams, lotions, pills, serums, and even surgical and non-surgical treatments that cater to those hoping to minimize or eliminate the appearance of wrinkles. Consumers spend billions of dollars annually purchasing these anti-wrinkle products. Assuming these products are safe, few consumers realize that the ingredients (many of which cannot easily be pronounced, let alone identified or understood by the general population) in these products can lead to serious skin conditions that result in far worse conditions than wrinkles.

Without the need for harsh applications or treatments, anyone hoping to minimize the appearance of wrinkles can combine a few simple, all-natural ingredients to create a natural wrinkle-reducing cream that can be used day or night for the prevention and reduction of wrinkles. While the results may not be visible for up to 2 weeks, the application will begin restoring the regenerative properties of the skin's cells immediately, including the collagen and elastin that helps improve skin elasticity and firmness for natural wrinkle elimination.

TO CREATE THIS ANTI-WRINKLE CREAM, FOLLOW THESE STEPS:

⅛ cup aloe vera
1 tablespoon vitamin E
1 tablespoon baking soda
2 tablespoons lemon juice

Combine the ingredients thoroughly by stirring them together in a small bowl.

Dab small amounts of the cream onto your face and then massage the treatment throughout the skin's surface. Rinse thoroughly with warm water.

87: MAKES A DIY DETOXIFYING MOISTURIZER

Many moisturizers promise to deliver the healthy glow, soft suppleness, and youthful appearance that so many strive to achieve. Consumers can choose from a wide variety of moisturizing products that claim to reduce wrinkles, correct discoloration, safeguard skin cell health, protect against harmful sun rays, or "reverse aging," but how often do you hear about these products detoxifying the skin?

The skin is the largest organ of the body, so it's surprising that a focus on promoting optimal skin health isn't emphasized more regularly by manufacturers of moisturizers. With the capability of seeping into the multiple layers of the skin, any topical treatment has the opportunity to affect the entire body's multiple intricate systems. This means that any moisturizer that is applied to the skin has the ability to deliver its chemicals, additives, and potential toxins directly into the bloodstream, transporting those elements throughout the body to every cell, organ, and system.

In order to avoid the toxic overload of the body's delicate components and essential processes, try an all-natural alternative that utilizes baking soda, aloe vera, coconut oil, and activated charcoal. With a combination of just 1 teaspoon of baking soda, ¼ teaspoon of activated charcoal powder, 1 tablespoon of aloe vera gel, and ¼ cup of coconut oil, you can create your very own DIY detoxifying moisturizer that can be applied as often as necessary for natural, effective relief. You'll find that the results are astounding! By absorbing toxins and toxic substances from the pores of the skin, the activated charcoal is able to remove harmful impurities naturally. The aloe vera and coconut oil not only moisturize the skin, but penetrate through deeper layers than most other moisturizers are capable of reaching. The baking soda's alkalizing effects combine with these ingredients to not only return the skin's pH to an optimal balance but also ensure that the healthy cells within the skin are able to retain their healthy membranes and perform as designed for the optimization of overall health throughout the skin's many layers.

88: MAKES A DETOXIFYING MAKEUP REMOVER

Countless cosmetic companies offer "permanent" makeups that promise to remain as applied throughout common situations such as weather, tears, and long periods of wear. While these options seem appealing to those who would rather not reapply and readjust their applications, these products can be difficult to remove when the day is done and there is no further want or need for the makeup to remain intact.

A laughable addition to "permanent" makeup applications are the makeup removal products that can "safely" remove the stains, smears, and smudges left behind from the countless assortments of makeup products that promise to stay in place for indefinite periods of time. Because these products often contain additives, chemicals, and questionable ingredients that can harm, irritate, and inflame the skin, many people are seeking out all-natural alternatives such a baking soda.

There are plenty of makeup remover products available that can be used on the areas of the skin and eyes where makeup is most commonly applied, but the safety of these products on the delicate areas of the face is up for debate. The chemical additions that must be used in these products to make them strong enough to remove "permanent" makeup with ease can have disastrous side effects. While ridding the face, lips, and eyes of the makeup that has been designed to stay put, these makeup removers can adversely affect the skin, resulting in redness, irritation, inflammation, peeling, and acne development.

When pursuing a safe, healthy makeup removal routine, the ultimate goal of safeguarding the skin should be first and foremost. The adage, "Nothing should be applied to your skin that you wouldn't feel safe enough eating," reminds us of the importance of our skin's permeability and the effects that topical applications can have on our bodies' internal workings. In place of these harsh consumer products, make your own makeup remover by simply combining 2 tablespoons of coconut oil and 1 tablespoon of baking soda. Soak a cotton ball in the mixture and then use it to gently remove any makeup while also moisturizing the skin and supporting the overall health of the body's skin and systems.

89: IMPROVES SKIN'S "GLOW"

One of the most delightful compliments a person can hear is that their skin "glows." With a radiance that exudes a sense of health, confidence, and beauty, the pursuit of the desirable glow has led many people to explore a number of possible products and procedures that promise to illuminate the skin. Whether these applications consist of makeup, bronzing dyes and sprays, or procedures that improve the circulation at the skin's surface, the most helpful pretreatment procedure would be one that includes baking soda.

Surprisingly, few people consider that the issue or condition that is most likely reducing the glowing appearance of skin is the buildup of dead skin cells, dirt, grime, and environmental toxins. While these elements are almost always present on the skin's surface as the body sheds dead cells, moves throughout multiple climate changes, and endures the ever-present hail of toxins and pollutants in the environment, the unnoticeable buildup can lead to a lackluster effect that can inhibit the skin's ability to shine with its healthiest appearance.

Luckily, baking soda can also be used in an all-natural skin treatment that can help remove buildup that blocks the "glow" of healthy skin with ease. Helping to regulate the pH balance of the skin, baking soda can not only improve skin's health but also assist in the gentle removal of film and deposits along its surface. By safely removing buildup without any damage to the skin's surface, this simple solution also helps alleviate or prevent the common conditions of irritation, inflammation, and redness that can jeopardize the skin's natural glow. By combining a simple solution of 2 tablespoons of lemon juice, 2 tablespoons of baking soda, ¼ cup of aloe vera, and ½ cup of all-natural sugar crystals, this rejuvenating body scrub can be applied over the skin's surface and massaged gently to remove impurities, dead skin cells, and toxins. In addition to the cleansing effect of this mildly abrasive combination, the soothing aloe and antioxidant-rich lemon juice help replenish the skin's natural moisture and vibrancy.

90: ACTS AS A GROWTH-PROMOTING NAIL SCRUB

With so many paints, soaks, washes, and pampering treatments designed to support nail health, it can be difficult to decide which is the best option for your unique nail health needs. As a general approach to the maintenance of nail health, the quality of the food you consume can play a major role. Adequate amounts of protein help provide the body with the strengthening "building blocks" that ensure nail growth and strength. In addition to a healthy diet, the daily nail hygiene and care of the surrounding skin can drastically impact the growth (or lack thereof) when it comes to nail health. By providing the nails with nutrient-rich, all-natural products that help remove dirt and grime while delivering strengthening support to the nails, nail beds, cuticles, and surrounding skin, nail health is protected and nail growth promoted.

In addition, with our nails being exposed to an unimaginable variety of germs, microbes, and toxins that lurk on every object and surface we touch throughout the day, it's no surprise that nail growth can be inhibited by even minor infections and irritations that may not even be noticeable to the naked eye. With the use of all-natural products such as 1 teaspoon of baking soda, 1 tablespoon of organic unfiltered apple cider vinegar, ¼ cup of Epsom salt, and ¼ cup of coconut oil, anyone hoping to strengthen their nails and promote nail growth naturally can find success with their own simple at-home concoction! With the replenishment of moisturizing, nutrient-rich aloe and coconut oil, enzyme-rich apple cider vinegar that combats harmful germs and microbes, baking soda that optimizes pH balance and alkalizes the tissue and gently cleanses nails, and Epsom salt that can naturally extract toxins, this simple concoction can be used to scrub nails free of dirt and germs while promoting the healthy, strong growth. Use this combination as a soak for 5–10 minutes daily and as a scrub that can be applied to the nails and nail beds with a gentle scrubbing action to remove dirt and grime healthfully.

91: REMEDIES AGE SPOTS

Age spots are the unsightly discolorations that appear on the skin's surface as we age. With these unsightly developments in the skin's normally uniform pigmentation, many age-spot sufferers turn to concealers or makeup in order to disguise the disruptions. With an increasingly large percentage of the population experiencing the development of these blemishes, the beauty industry has responded with multiple treatment options that promise to minimize the size, color, or number of age spots that can occur throughout the skin's surface. While many of these products seem promising, they rarely rid the skin of the discolored areas. By choosing to provide the body with all-natural remedies that are intended to treat the underlying causes, the body's systems can work in harmony to correct certain deficiencies or disruptions. These natural treatment methods also include topical applications that can be applied to affected areas of the skin, helping to minimize the appearance of the discolored areas as well.

Baking soda has an outstanding effect on skin conditions by promoting the proper pH balance of the skin's surface, improving the body's natural shedding of dead skin cells, and maximizing the proper processing of nutrients that can improve skin health. With the daily ingestion of 1 tablespoon of baking soda dissolved in an 8-ounce glass of water, the body's natural pH can be returned to an optimal alkaline state in which all systems function as intended. With this optimized functioning, the entire body becomes better able to process nutrients and experience benefits. When the skin receives the dietary nutrients and hydration it needs, minor conditions, such as age spots, can be diminished naturally over time. In addition, a spot-treatment consisting of 1 tablespoon of baking soda and 1 tablespoon of water can be applied to afflicted areas for 15-minute periods three times daily for visible improvements in as little as 2–4 weeks.

92: COMBATS CANCEROUS SKIN CHANGES

Throughout life, the cells of the body undergo countless changes and transformations. While these changes are naturally intended to support the life cycle by optimizing the functioning of the organs and systems, there are times when cellular changes can be unhealthy. With exposure to toxic substances, environmental hazards, and other situations that can interfere with the proper functioning of cells, carcinogenic changes can occur. One of the most prominent areas of the body that experiences these unhealthy transformations is the skin. With the skin being regularly exposed to toxins in the environment, sunlight, and even organic compounds that can be absorbed directly through the skin's sensitive layers, cancerous skin changes can occur in many diverse populations regardless of their location or lifestyle habits. While some experiences can make the development of these dangerous changes more likely, anyone is at risk of succumbing to skin cancer.

By incorporating baking soda into an everyday routine, the average person can help minimize the risk of cancerous changes in skin cells. With the daily ingestion of 1 tablespoon of baking soda dissolved in an 8-ounce glass of water, the alkalizing benefits combat the acidity in the body that contributes to the cancerous development and growth. With the added benefit of a baking soda–based topical paste made of 1 part baking soda and 1 part aloe vera, the skin's surface absorbs the very elements and nutrients that can safeguard cells within the skin from carcinogenic activity. Prior to rinsing the application, the nutrients not only absorb into the skin, but help retain in the skin's cells so they can be utilized for healthy processes such as cell protection, skin cell regeneration, and antiaging. With this simple two-step approach to healing the internal and external aspects of the body's sensitive cells, you can minimize your risk of skin cancer while maximizing your overall health naturally.

93: MENDS SPLIT ENDS

Wet hair's open cuticles and strands become exposed to chemical-containing shampoos, conditioners, and treatments, and then brushes, combs, and blow-outs continue the damage to your hair's health. There are countless products that promise to provide protection for your hair, and it can be easy to try these heavily marketed "solutions," but baking soda can actually offer protections naturally.

Every year, consumers spend trillions of dollars on hair care products and treatments that are intended to preserve the natural beauty of luscious locks. While these products can provide countless benefits, such as adding volume, reducing frizz, accentuating color and highlights, and preserving the health of each strand, the legitimacy of products that claim to be able to repair split ends remains up for debate. While it is true that a hair strand that has split cannot be re-fused or repaired, the mending process can be effective when precautionary measures are taken to preserve the integrity of and promote the health of the hair. Through research and extensive experimentation, it has been determined that certain treatments (such as excessive coloring or styling with heat), certain environmental conditions (such as exposure to pollution or extremely drying conditions), and even styling procedures (such as brushing hair while wet or consistently wearing hair styled by abrasive materials such as elastic) can all degrade the strength of hair strands, making them more susceptible to damage. By avoiding these dangers and implementing a regular baking soda application, anyone can mend their hair and prevent split ends.

A combination of ½ cup of baking soda and 1 cup of coconut oil creates a hair mask that rejuvenates hair strands, balances pH, and moisturizes the scalp and follicles. This treatment can be applied to dry hair for a period of 20 minutes and rinsed thoroughly up to three times weekly for healthier hair that can withstand the risks posed by everyday maintenance and activities safely, easily, and beautifully.

94: MAKES A DRY SHAMPOO

Years ago, many hairstylists and consumers started to take notice of the adverse effects regular shampooing and conditioning was having on even the healthiest heads of hair. With a little research and experimentation, it was determined that the ingredients that shampoos contain to remove dirt and grime from the scalp and strands can actually be detrimental to the natural makeup of the hair as well as the hair's health and appearance. One area of major concern is that excessive hair washing can rid the scalp and strands of essential oils that are released to ensure that moisture is retained throughout. When these oils are consistently stripped from the scalp and hair, the result is a rebound effect in which the glands overcompensate and overproduce the oils that were simply intended to maintain optimal health.

In order to ensure that the essential oil production for healthy hair remains in a natural balance, many consumers have opted for a minimal hair washing routine that limits shampoo applications to once or twice weekly, if at all. The result of this avoidance of shampoo treatments includes an initial experience of oily or greasy strands, but this is quickly followed by a return to optimal oil production that leaves hair looking and feeling healthier than ever. While this transition from the texture and appearance of regularly shampooed hair to the greasier alternative once shampooing is discontinued can be difficult or uncomfortable, there is an all-natural approach that can help rid the hair of greasiness while still promoting the hair and scalp's optimal health: baking soda!

By applying $\frac{1}{8}$–$\frac{1}{4}$ cup of baking soda to the hair, this naturally alkalizing ingredient helps dry excessive oils while also improving the hair's pH balance. Making an effort to avoid applying the baking soda directly to the scalp, simply flip hair upside down and sprinkle the baking soda throughout the strands and toward the base of the roots. Brush the baking soda through the hair and reveal the outstanding results of a dry shampoo that not only leaves your hair looking and feeling great but smelling fresh and clean too!

95: MAKES A VOLUMIZING SHAMPOO

There is a seemingly endless supply of shampoo products available to consumers, making it difficult to decipher which option is the right choice for your hair's needs. Whether you have bone-straight hair that won't comply with any volumizing product's promises or curly hair that won't be tamed by any tress-teasing tousle, the battle to find the perfect median for your own type of hair can be hard. Marketing companies spend billions of dollars every year trying to appeal to "you" for good reason. There are shampoos that promise to promote shine, curls, bounce, and frizz-free hair among countless other aesthetically appealing results, causing your shampoo selection to become a daunting endeavor. When it comes to choosing the perfect application or treatment for volumizing effects on hair, though, there are a number of factors to take into consideration. With many shampoos containing harsh chemicals and additives such as sulfates, parabens, and even potent fragrances, these ingredients can often leave your hair dry, brittle, and damaged rather than full of voluminous body.

Luckily, baking soda makes for the perfect volumizing shampoo with health benefits galore! With the ability to remove dirt, oil, grime, and buildup, a baking soda–based rinse can be used to safely cleanse the hair's strands of the very elements that weigh it down and restrict your hair's voluminous appearance. In addition to removing the heavy compounds that can gradually build up over time and flatten hair, this baking soda solution can improve hair health, rid the scalp of dandruff, and help restore shine to strands. Simply combine 1 part baking soda and 3 parts water. Then apply the solution to wet hair by pouring the rinse over the head to saturate the hair, gently massaging the scalp to ensures that the hair is soaked thoroughly. Let the solution set on the hair for 1–3 minutes before rinsing with cold water and conditioning as usual.

96: REMOVES HAIR-PRODUCT BUILDUP

If you feel your hair falling flat, feeling greasy, looking oily, or not responding well to normal treatments, the issue may be as simple as common product buildup. One of the most common complaints in terms of hair care, treatments, styling, and procedures is the gradual buildup of residue that can be left behind on strands. The variety of products consumers use for styling, adding shine, smoothing frizz, adding volume, increasing elasticity in curls, and straightening hair all leave slight layers of film and residue that can build up even with regular washing and rinsing. Many people don't realize that this buildup is often the cause of their hair's lackluster appearance, and that it can inhibit a product's desired effect on the hair—even interfering with the optimal growth of the hair and health of the scalp. While countless products promise to remove hair-product buildup without compromising the composition of the strands or producing adverse reactions, many of the options out there contain harsh chemicals that can strip the proteins from hair and leave weak, lackluster hair prone to damage or breakage.

By utilizing a leave-in, baking soda–based paste made of 1 cup of water and 1 cup of baking soda, you can apply the paste to the strands of your hair and reap its alkalizing, pH-balancing benefits as it neutralizes acidity and breaks down dirt, grime, and buildup without causing any damage to hair. Simply make the paste, apply it to your scalp, and massage it throughout the hair. Leave the paste in the hair for 3–5 minutes before rinsing. Following the use of this treatment, you can condition your hair and style normally without the cumbersome weight of old product residue that had been hiding your hair's true beauty all along!

97: REJUVENATES OILY HAIR

Oily hair is one of the most common complaints among people hoping to achieve flawless locks that can be styled to last throughout the day. When the hair's natural oil balance is disrupted, the result can be unsightly oil deposits that not only become obvious on the crown of the head but can also lead to excessive dryness at the ends of your strands. This oily hair condition can be remedied by a number of available products designed to dry the scalp and rid the hair of oils, but these products can also contain harsh chemicals and additives that may cause more harm than good.

Baking soda has been used as an effective remedy for oily hair conditions for years, and it has been well documented as an effective solution for not just excessive oil but also preventing future oily buildup. By using the dry shampoo recipe (listed in entry 94), you can apply a generous amount of baking soda to the roots and strands of the hair before brushing. Not only can the baking soda counteract the oils and buildup that contribute to a greasy appearance, this treatment helps restore an optimal pH balance that aids in healthy levels of oil production and won't leave a greasy residue behind. You can also create a baking soda–based in-shower conditioning mask by adding 1 tablespoon of baking soda to your favorite conditioner to combat acidity.

Ingesting 1 tablespoon of baking soda dissolved in an 8-ounce glass of water can also help regulate the hormones and systems involved in oil production to ensure that the situation resolves by simply correcting internal issues you may not have previously considered.

98: REMEDIES CHLORINATED "SWIMMERS' HAIR"

Swimmers who regularly engage in underwater activities reap countless benefits to the circulatory and skeletal systems, muscles, metabolism, and even cognitive functioning and mental focus. This low-impact activity that provides immense health benefits has inspired a rising number of fitness-focused individuals to include swimming in their regular exercise routines. While the list of physical benefits is exhaustive, swimming in chlorinated pools can have one adverse effect: swimmer's hair. Over-chlorination and overuse of chemicals common in pool water can do catastrophic damage to hair.

Each strand of hair contains pores that quickly absorb any liquid it comes in contact with, including chlorinated pool water. Once chlorine infiltrates the hair, exposure to heavy metals such as copper, iron, and magnesium can create an oxidizing interaction, which results in hair that appears green. In addition to the new hue, chlorine exposure can lead to excessively dry hair, flyaways, and even brittle ends. There are a number of products that promise to provide swimmers with protection against these adverse effects, but many fail to work and most contain chemicals and unsafe additives that can exacerbate existing hair issues.

With a baking soda rinse comprised of 1 part baking soda and 3 parts water, a swimmer can douse her hair before entering the pool for a safeguard against chlorine and heavy metal interactions inside the hair's pores. Following a swim, if the swimmer notices significant color changes in her hair, a baking soda–based paste made of 1 part baking soda and 1 part water can be applied throughout the affected strands and allowed to set for 5 minutes. Afterward the treatment should be rinsed thoroughly and followed up with a regular conditioning treatment.

99: DISINFECTS COMBS AND BRUSHES

While the dishes, floors, bathrooms, bedding, and laundry all get ample attention when it comes to maintaining a healthy home, there are a few regularly used items that rarely receive the attention they deserve. In the processes of styling hair every day, few people realize that their hair brushes and combs come into contact with dead skin cells from the scalp, dry skin flakes, oils, dirt, grime, and deposits of hair product residue that can build up on the bristles and teeth of these hair care tools. While styling tools may not seem hazardous, there's a real possibility of bacteria breeding among the flat surfaces and bristles, which can be deposited throughout the hair while coming into direct contact with the scalp, and from there the microbes can seep directly into the bloodstream and create complications for the brain, blood, cells, organs, and other bodily systems.

In an effort to maintain safe, clean hair tools, it is imperative that you clean brushes and combs regularly. Rather than using harsh rinses that contain chemicals and unsafe ingredients that could adversely affect hair strands and irritate the scalp, baking soda can be used to break down residual oils and deposits on brushes and combs, restoring a positive pH balance to the hair the next time it comes in contact with those styling tools.

Create a solution of 1 part baking soda and 3 parts water. Once all hair and obvious particles have been removed from the brushes and combs, submerge the hair tools in the solution and allow them to soak for 60 minutes. Dry the tools with a hair dryer, and repeat this cleansing process at least once per month.

100: MAKES A COLOR-SECURING HAIR RINSE

Whether it's for a special occasion or just to combat gray hairs, many consumers seek out new and exciting ways to preserve the hair colors and highlights that they love. Even for those who choose to retain their natural hair color, there is a constant awareness that the color can quickly change when it's exposed to extensive sunlight, other weather conditions, or chlorine and minerals common in swimming pools. Multiple beauty product manufacturers have created protective powders, creams, rinses, shampoos, and conditioners that promise to safeguard individuals' hair colors. As with so many manufactured products, though, many of these color-preserving treatments contain caustic chemicals and additives that can adversely affect the health of the hair or possibly adversely interact with the hair's color.

Baking soda has an alkalizing benefit that helps return the pH to a more neutral, healthy state by eroding and negating harsh chemicals, minerals, and elements. It's this feature, that makes it an ideal solution for preserving any kind of hair color—from natural and artificial to sun-bleached. And best of all, it doesn't interact with or change the color of hair it comes in contact with. By using a baking soda rinse (listed in entry 98), the application of baking soda–based dry shampoo (listed in entry 94), and baking soda–based pastes (listed in entry 98), there are a number of baking soda treatments that not only rid the hair of buildup, chemicals, and minerals that can transform hair color but also work proactively to improve the health of hair strands and the scalp to ensure that damage doesn't occur and will not continue to occur.

INDEX

A

Acidity, reducing. *See* pH

Acne. *See* Skin care

Age spots, remedying, 105

Allergies, easing, 36

Aloe vera

beauty benefits, 70

for cancerous skin
changes, 106

for detoxifying moisturizer,
101

detoxifying pores, 87

for diaper rash, 75

exfoliating skin with, 74

for face cleanser, 83

for face mask, 84

for footbath, 77

for hand soap, 85

for immunity, 16

for insect bites, 23

for natural pet rinse, 61

for rashes, 71

for razor burn, 96

scrubs with, 88, 98, 104

skin benefits, 20, 70, 103

soothing lotion with, 70

for sunburns, 69

for tattoo applications, 99

for wrinkle reduction,
100

Aluminum, baking soda and, 11

Antacid. *See* Digestion

Arthritis, minimizing, 19

B

Baking soda. *See also specific uses*

aluminum misconception, 11

benefits overview, 9, 11–12

history of, 10–11

how to use, 11–12

pH of, 10

range of uses, 7

safety precautions, 12

scientific (chemical) names, 10

this book and, 7

what it is, 10

Banana smoothie, antacid-alternative, 56

Baths, baking soda

dry, for pets, 60

for irritated skin, 73

for migraines, 47

natural pet rinse, 61

removing spray/fake tan, 89

as skunk deodorizer, 59

soothing footbath, 76, 77

for sunburns, 69

Beauty uses, overview of, 67. *See also Skin references; specific topics*

D

E

F

pre-manicure treatment, 80
removing yellowing/stains
from, 79
Nervous system
improving functioning of,
21
pH balance and, 21, 44

O

Odors, removing. *See* Deodorants
Oily hair, rejuvenating, 111
Oily skin, mask for, 84
Oral health. *See also* Breath, bad,
treating
cleansing mouth devices (dentures,
retainers, etc.), 31
of dogs and cats. *See* Pets
kid-safe cavity-fighting mouth
rinse, 93
natural mouthwash, 92
natural toothpaste, 90
overnight soak solution, 31
plaque removal, 95
soothing sore teeth and gums,
49
whitening teeth, 91
Orange juice, reducing acidity of,
53

P

Parasites, combatting/treating, 40
Pets
accidents, treating, 62
bad breath treatment, 66
bleeding-nail treatment, 65
cleansing teeth and gums, 63
deodorizing, cleaning litterboxes, 64
dog-sweat smell deodorant, 60
dry bath for, 60
natural rinse for, 61
relieving insect bites, 23
pH
about: of baking soda, 10
antacid from baking soda, 32
balancing, 14, 18, 44, 50
nervous system functioning and, 21
reducing acidity of orange juice, 53
smoothie for balancing, 50
yeast infections and, 37
Plaque, removing, 95
Pores, detoxifying, 97
Produce, removing residue from, 58

R

Rashes, relieving, 71, 75. *See also* Skin
irritation/issues
Razor burn, soothing, 96

Rehydrating body, 38

Reparation, exercise, 28

Reproductive health
  improving, 22
  UTI treatment and, 46
  yeast infections and, 37

Residue on produce, removing, 58

Respiratory system. *See also* Coughs,
    colds, and flu
  baking soda benefits, 17
  functions of, 17
  improving airway functioning, 17
  killing fungi, mildew, mold
      and, 39

Retainers, cleansing, 31

S

Safety precautions, 12

Salad, kale, for cleansing, 57

Scientific (chemical) names, 10

Scrubs
  for brightening skin, 88
  exfoliating scrub, 74
  growth-promoting nail
      scrub, 104
  improving skin's "glow," 103
  moisturizing facial scrub, 98
  therapeutic body scrub, 78

Shampoo. *See* Hair care; Pets

Skeletal system, baking soda
    benefits, 18

Skin care. *See also* Hair care; Nails;
    Scrubs
  acne spot treatment, 82
  age spot remedy, 105
  blackhead remedy, 87
  brightening skin, 88
  detoxifying makeup
      remover, 102
  detoxifying moisturizer, 101
  detoxifying pores, 97
  exfoliating skin, 74
  face cleanser, 83
  face mask for oily skin, 84
  hand soap, 85
  hand-softening lotion, 70
  improving skin's "glow,"
      103
  reducing wrinkles, 100
  removing spray/fake tan, 89
  softening calluses, 81
  softening feet, 76
  soothing footbath, 77
  soothing razor burn, 96

Skin irritation/issues
  cancerous skin changes, 106
  chicken pox irritations, alleviating, 30
  diaper rash treatment, 75

ABOUT THE AUTHOR

Britt Brandon is a certified personal trainer and certified fitness nutrition specialist (certified by the International Sports Sciences Association, ISSA) and health coach (certified by the American Council on Exercise, ACE) who has enjoyed writing books that focus on clean eating, fitness, and unique health-promoting ingredients such as apple cider vinegar, coconut oil, and aloe vera for Adams Media. In her time with Adams, she has published eleven books, including *The Everything® Green Smoothies Book*, *The Everything® Eating Clean Cookbook*, *What Color Is Your Smoothie?*, *The Everything® Eating Clean Cookbook for Vegetarians*, *The Everything® Healthy Green Drinks Book*, and *The Everything® Guide to Pregnancy Nutrition & Health*. As a competitive athlete, trainer, mom of three small children, and fitness and nutrition blogger on her own website (UltimateFitMom.com), she is well versed in the holistic approaches to keeping oneself in top performing condition.